<7 C0 AGD5578>

Curriculum for Educators in Health Care Institutions

Proceedings and Recommendations of an Invitational Conference

by
Patty L. Dunkel

Hospital Research and Educational Trust
840 North Lake Shore Drive • Chicago, Illinois 60611

Library of Congress Cataloging in Publication Data

Main entry under title:

Curriculum for educators in health care institutions.

    SUMMARY of the proceedings of a conference held on
January 6-7, 1977.
    1. Hospitals—Staff—In-service training—Congresses
2. Hospitals—Staff—In-service training—Teacher
training—Congresses. I. Dunkel, Patty L.,
1930-   II. Hospital Research Educational Trust.
[DNLM: 1. Curriculum—Congresses. 2. Health
occupations—Education—Congresses. 3. Inservice
training—Congresses. W18 D919c 1977]
RA972.5.C87   610′.7′15   77-26933
ISBN 0-87914-046-1

HRET Catalog Number: 9620

© 1978 by the
Hospital Research and Educational Trust
840 North Lake Shore Drive
Chicago, Illinois 60611

HRET T-46

3M—2/78—462

10/12 Times Roman and Optima

Contents

PREFACE   v

PARTICIPANTS   vii

STAFF   ix

INTRODUCTION   1

WELCOMING REMARKS   3

PERSPECTIVES ON EDUCATORS AND EDUCATION
IN HEALTH CARE INSTITUTIONS   5

Administrator's View of the Director of Education   5

Director's View of the Education Staff   6

The Scope of Education in the Hospital   8

Findings of a Functional Job Analysis   11

Findings of the Hospitalwide Education
and Training Project   15

Guidelines on Developing Curriculum   19

CURRICULAR RECOMMENDATIONS   21

Preservice Nondegree Program   21

Inservice Nondegree Program   25

Degree Program   27

SUMMARY   33

Recommendations on Future Activities   35

Closing Remarks   36

APPENDIX A.   Glossary   37

APPENDIX B.   A Functional Job Analysis of Educators
in Health Care Institutions: Implications
for Higher and Continuing
Education Curriculums   39

APPENDIX C.   Questionnaire for Health Manpower
Educators and Trainers   69

Preface

An invitational conference on curriculum for educators in health care institutions was held in Chicago at the Hospital Research and Educational Trust, an affiliate of the American Hospital Association, on January 6-7, 1977. Its purpose was to explore the nature of education and training in health care institutions and to develop recommendations for curriculums for persons working or wishing to work in this field. The conference was conducted by staff of the Trust's Hospitalwide Education and Training Project (HETP), a five-year demonstration project funded by a grant from the W. K. Kellogg Foundation, Battle Creek, MI.

Invitations were extended to 27 representatives of programs that were directed to or that had potential responsibility for the education of educators in health care institutions. Twenty-two of these attended the conference, 20 from the United States and 2 from Canada. The participants represented college and university programs in adult education, hospital administration, and nursing; divisions of university extensions; hospital departments of education and training; and the American Society for Health Manpower Education and Training (ASHET), a personal membership society of the AHA. Also attending were five members of the HETP staff and one member of the AHA's Department of Education.

A planning committee of prospective participants met in December 1976 to advise HETP staff on the program for the conference. Because of the widely varying backgrounds of the participants, the committee recommended that a series of lectures and discussions be provided to explicate the different assumptions held by individual participants about education in health care institutions and that a glossary be compiled and distributed to participants before the conference.

The committee also suggested that the curricular recommendations to be developed meet two criteria: they should be readily adaptable to the wide variety of organizational settings in which education was being pro-

v

vided for hospital educators and they should take into account the issue of academic freedom. The members agreed that a series of competency statements, each including a description of expected learner behavior and of content or subject matter, would meet the two criteria. They also approved a suggestion that three sets of curricular recommendations be developed: one for preservice nondegree programs, one for inservice nondegree programs, and one for degree programs. Definitions of these programs are given in Appendix A.

The HETP staff did not think it expedient to present a verbatim transcript of the proceedings of the conference. What is presented in these pages is a summary of the deliberations and recommendations made by the participants, including some of the concerns that they faced in developing curriculums. Lectures given on the first day of the conference have been summarized, followed by highlights of the discussions that ensued. Because much of the conference was devoted to the activities of small work groups, the reports of these groups and the related discussions also have been summarized. The author takes full responsibility for any omissions in the final text.

A conference of this type depends on the efforts of many persons. Without the generous support of the W. K. Kellogg Foundation, the conference would not have been possible. Grateful acknowledgment also is extended to the members of the planning committee, who gave of their time and talent in advising the HETP staff.

The proceedings themselves are much richer for the thoughtful comments of Bob Munk, Marc Lovett, and Dianne Spenner, and without the first draft, which was written by Ann Ogden, the proceedings would not exist. A special note of thanks is extended to Ms. Spenner, who handled the many details of conference administration with deftness, and to Patricia Martin, who typed the final draft of these proceedings.

PATTY L. DUNKEL
Conference Coordinator

Participants

George F. Aker
Professor of Adult Education
Florida State University
Tallahassee, FL

John C. Booth
Assistant Professor and
    Coordinator
Health Services Management
    Program
School of Allied Health
Ferris State College
Big Rapids, MI

James A. Brigham*
Chairman
Department of Hospital and
    Health Care Administration
St. Louis University
St. Louis, MO

H. Walton Connelly*
Director of Education and
    Training
Methodist Hospital of Indiana
Indianapolis, IN

Alan G. Cotzin
Director of Education and
    Training
Bay State Medical Center
Springfield, MA

Margaret E. Courtney
Director of Continuing Education
    in Nursing
Evening College
Johns Hopkins University
Baltimore, MD

David R. Day
Professor of Organizational
    Behavior
Sangamon State University
Springfield, IL

Nancy Diekelmann
Associate Professor
School of Nursing
University of Wisconsin
Madison, WI

---

*Member of the planning committee, which also included Robert L. Finkelmeier, director, Personnel and Training Service, University of Colorado Medical Center, Denver

William S. Griffith*
Associate Professor and Chairman
Committee on Educational Design
    and Implementation
Department of Education
University of Chicago
Chicago, IL

Howard W. Houser
Department Chairman and
    Associate Professor
Graduate Program in Hospital
    and Health Administration
University of Alabama in
    Birmingham
Birmingham, AL

Rose Kennedy
Director
American Society for Health
    Manpower Education and
    Training
American Hospital Association
Chicago, IL

Barbara Knudson
Dean
University College
University of Minnesota
Minneapolis, MN

Frank Malouff
Training Administrator
University of Colorado Medical
    Center
Denver, CO

Barbara P. McCool*
Associate Professor
Department of Health
    Administration
Duke University
Durham, NC

Herman Mullins
Associate Professor
School of Allied Health
    Professions
Virginia Commonwealth
    University
Richmond, VA

Leonard Nadler*
Professor
Adult Education and Human
    Resources Development
George Washington University
Washington, DC

Barbara Nichols
Director
Hospitalwide Inservice Education
St. Mary's Hospital Medical
    Center
Madison, WI

Donald Sanders
Professor of Education
Ohio State University
Columbus, OH

*Member of the planning committee

Robert Shouldice
Assistant Professor
School of Government and
    Business Administration
George Washington University
Washington, DC

Alan Thomas
Chairman
Department of Adult Education
Ontario Institute for Studies in
    Education
Toronto, Ontario, Canada

Coolie Verner
Chairman
Department of Adult Education
University of British Columbia
Vancouver, BC, Canada

George R. Wren
Director and Professor
Institute of Health Administration
Georgia State University
Atlanta, GA

Staff

Jeffrey Butler
Educational Design Specialist
Department of Education
American Hospital Association

Patty L. Dunkel
Research Associate
Hospitalwide Education and
    Training Project
Hospital Research and
    Educational Trust

Herbert K. Gatzke
Project Administrator
Hospitalwide Education and
    Training Project

Marc Lovett
Project Director
Hospitalwide Education and
    Training Project

Robert J. Munk
Research Associate
Hospitalwide Education and
    Training Project

Dianne V. Spenner
Project Assistant
Hospitalwide Education and
    Training Project

INTRODUCTION

The two-day conference on curriculum for educators in health care institutions opened with general sessions designed to provide background information for the participants. Staff of the Hospitalwide Education and Training Project (HETP) described the history and goals of the project and explained how the conference was to contribute to meeting those goals. They also described the nature of the curricular recommendations that were to be developed during the course of the conference.

Three speakers, who had been selected from among the participants, examined educators and education in the hospital from different perspectives. Following these lectures and the discussions related to them, two members of the HETP staff summarized and led discussions of papers that they had written under the project and had distributed to participants prior to the conference.

The final speaker in these sessions presented a series of guidelines to assist the work groups in developing their curricular recommendations for preservice nondegree programs, inservice nondegree programs, and degree programs. Participants then divided into three work groups, each of which was responsible for developing curricular recommendations for one of the three types of educational programs. Each participant selected a group on the basis of individual interest and professional background. The reports of the work groups were presented and discussed on the second day of the conference.

1

WELCOMING REMARKS

In his welcome to the group, Herbert K. Gatzke, manager, Division of Management Effectiveness, AHA, and project administrator, HETP, outlined the context in which the conference was occurring. "Back as far as 1964, the W. K. Kellogg Foundation gave a sizable grant to the Hospital Research and Educational Trust for the Hospital Continuing Education Project." One of the basic thrusts of this project, Mr. Gatzke said, was to stimulate hospitals to develop and maintain competent health manpower through hospitalwide education and training. Another was to work with seven major universities to establish continuing education centers for health care personnel. A number of these centers still are operating, he noted.

As a result of 18 conferences that were held during the course of the project, "a new profession began to emerge, called 'hospital training director' or 'hospital education director.' In 1970, the American Society for Health Manpower Education and Training was formed within the AHA, and it now has about 1,250 members."

When the project ended in 1972, Mr. Gatzke continued, the Kellogg Foundation provided support to the Trust for a second education project, the Hospitalwide Education and Training Project. "Its primary objective was to demonstrate different models of organization, to ask, 'How is the education and training function organized in the hospital?' 'How does it relate to other aspects of the hospital structure?' and 'What impact do these different organizational models have on the effectiveness or the success of the function in the institution?'

"The second purpose of the HETP was to look at the tasks performed by the persons who carry on this function, to define the skills that these persons need, and, eventually, to make recommendations concerning the kinds of preparation, either in degree programs or short courses, that would help directors of education to develop these skills.

"That is the part of the project with which you are most directly concerned. In the time available, I do not assume that you will come out with a polished product. I do expect that we will have had the benefit of your experience in curriculum development and that we will have enough detailed information with which to fashion a set of observations and recommendations on some actions that should be taken in the future," Mr. Gatzke said.

Expectations for the Conference

Patty L. Dunkel, research associate, HETP, elaborated on the structure of the recommendations that were expected to emerge from the conference: "Separate work groups will develop recommendations for curriculum for preservice nondegree programs, inservice nondegree programs, and degree programs. Each recommendation should include both a behavioral component and a subject matter component. Otherwise, we are placing no limitations on the kinds of statements that you develop."

She also called attention to the definition that would be used throughout the conference for the terms *educator* and *trainer:* the professional who has responsibility for the education, training, and development of persons who work in hospitals or who are patients in them.

PERSPECTIVES ON EDUCATORS AND EDUCATION IN HEALTH CARE INSTITUTIONS

Administrator's View of the Director of Education

The perspective of the administrator on the position of director of education was presented by James A. Brigham Jr., formerly a hospital administrator and currently chairman, department of hospital and health care administration, St. Louis University, St. Louis, MO. Mr. Brigham had consulted with a number of hospital administrators to obtain their thoughts about the role and qualifications of a director of education.

The administrator, Mr. Brigham said, sees the director of education both as a staff specialist and as a manager with line responsibilities. Mr. Brigham identified five abilities that administrators commonly view as being crucial to the director's role as a staff resource. These abilities are as follows:

- To develop organizational policy with respect to education.
- To assist in problem-solving. The unique role that the director of education plays is to point out when education can serve in solving organizational problems.
- To serve as a mediator between those persons within the hospital who define patient care as the hospital's primary function and those who define education as the primary function.
- To serve as a mediator between the hospital and educational institutions, that is, to screen the demands that external institutions place on the hospital to provide clinical experiences. As examples of such kinds of experiences that hospitals are providing, Mr. Brigham cited programs for community college law enforcement aides, social work aides, laboratory aides, home health aides, and dental aides. "It gets to be expensive and time

5

consuming, and somehow there has to be some arbitration," he said.

- To justify to third-party payers and the general public the costs of education in terms of its contribution to patient care. However, Mr. Brigham cautioned against becoming so concerned with justifying costs incurred that possibilities for cost reductions would be overlooked.

Turning to the qualifications that administrators look for in a director of education, he noted "the wide variety of persons currently serving in this role." However, he identified some common expectations held by administrators for persons in the position. He placed these qualifications in three categories:

- Skills in managing and sensitivity to people and resources. "There was surprising emphasis on management ability," Mr. Brigham said.
- Sensitivity to and knowledge of issues and problems in health care, especially the social organization of the health care institution and the values that are associated with the provision of services.
- Sensitivity to and skills in administering educational programs in a health care setting.

A participant suggested that administrators, despite their ideas about the staff specialist role, appear to look primarily for a good manager. "Do they really know how they want to use this person?" he asked.

Mr. Brigham responded that the role of staff specialist in hospitals is new, especially the specialist in education. Consequently, he said, administrators tend to look for persons with management skills because they are more familiar with management selection criteria.

Director's View of the Education Staff

Presenting the perspective of a director of education on selecting education staff members, Frank Malouff, training administrator, University of Colorado Medical Center, Denver, said, "Some of the characteristics that I look for in a person for the training staff are some of the ones that I would look for in a manager."

The six characteristics that he cited are as follows:

- The ability to motivate. "I look for a leader, a slightly Machiavellian person."

- The ability to communicate, which includes the ability to listen. "The trainer has to be a problem-spotter, a problem-solver, and an evaluator," Mr. Malouff said. "Further, the trainer should be nonthreatening, empathetic, and patient; should collaborate with others; and should be a resource, not an authority," he added.
- The potential to be a facilitator. Mr. Malouff explained that the trainer must be capable of integrating the goals and activities of the education department with the overall goals of the organization.
- An instinctive understanding of the environment and of the ethics of the institution and a willingness to be an advocate for the institution.
- The ability to be an agent of change. He said that the staff must be ready for change, "must be ahead of it, if you will. The staff must be able to look ahead." As an example of the need for this characteristic, he cited the trend toward increasing numbers of malpractice suits being filed against hospitals. There have been cases, he said, in which the staff directly affected the outcome of malpractice suits. "What is the role of teaching risk management?" he asked.
- A little bit of the "entertainer" ego.

"Some of these characteristics are teachable, others are not. I do not believe that you can find all six in one person," Mr. Malouff commented.

Following Mr. Malouff's presentation, a representative of a university program in health administration pointed out that knowledge about and skills in education had not been mentioned, and he asked, "Was that intentional?"

A representative of a continuing education program in nursing added, "If all that you are concerned about are managerial skills, then why are we here? What is the difference between the curriculum for the hospital administrator and that for the training director?"

Mr. Malouff replied, "I do not downgrade educational skills, but most applicants have some background in education. I would like to emphasize that, from a very practical point of view, I am more concerned about finding staff members with certain unteachable characteristics than with backgrounds in education."

An adult educationist said, "Some characteristics, while they may be learned, may not be teachable in the usual sense of the word 'teachable.'

I'm interested, however, in the characteristics that you think are teachable and in those that you think are not teachable. There is a body of knowledge in adult education that covers many of the characteristics that you think are unteachable. For example, if you had a trained educator, you would not be looking for an 'entertainer' or a Machiavelli."

The Scope of Education in the Hospital

H. Walton Connelly, director of education and training, Methodist Hospital of Indiana, Indianapolis, focused the participants' attention on the scope of educational programs being conducted in hospitals. Mr. Connelly stated that he was "thoroughly convinced" that hospital administrators had a limited notion of the amount of education currently being conducted in the hospital and of the possibilities for improving this education. "Adult educators have yet to recognize the potential that is available in the social organization that we call the hospital," he said.

Looking at the current situation, he described several categories of hospital education and training, beginning with preservice programs. "The hospital is unusual," he said, "because of the amount of preservice training that it requires for its employees. For example, a department store can train someone to work the cash register and to maintain the store's computerized inventory control in about seven hours, but the hospital rarely places anyone in an entry-level position after just seven hours of training." The enormous amount of preservice training that has to be conducted, he continued, is necessary for the survival of the organization. "It is necessary if the organization is to exist in 1978."

Inservice training, the second category, "is the type that is most accepted," said Mr. Connelly. "Obviously, preservice training is conducted before a person takes a position, and inservice training is done so that the employee can perform more effectively the job that he already holds."

The third category of educational activity is upgrading, that is, training "designed to allow a person to move into a position that is a step or two higher in job classification. In this area, the hospital is unusual in that career ladders and career lattices are almost nonexistent," he stated. "In my view, this causes serious personnel problems. Hospitals are trying to remedy this situation by developing some career ladders and lattices and by providing related education and training for employees."

The fourth category is continuing education. Because of the variety of professions within the hospital, Mr. Connelly said, "there is a great struggle for status and identity. In my view, continuing education has become a part of that struggle. What the hospital educator needs to do is to use this struggle to help members of the various occupational groups to become more competent in their fields."

The fifth category that Mr. Connelly identified is management and supervisory training, which he said is becoming increasingly important. Managers in hospitals "need to come from the professional groups. They have been well trained in their own technologies but have not been trained in management," he pointed out.

Enrichment training, the sixth category, is a result of the "move up in expectations" for job satisfaction through such fringe benefits as educational opportunities. "The hospital, as a major employer in most communities, is beginning to recognize the need and the opportunity for enrichment training," he said.

Health education is just beginning to emerge as a category of hospital education and eventually will overshadow all of the others, Mr. Connelly predicted. Within this category, he identified three target groups: employees, members of the community, and patients. Regarding the latter group, he foresees the physician ordering education for patients as part of the treatment plan. "Theoretically, we ought to have a moment for teaching with each new patient, but the problem is that we do not know what to do in that situation. We have done very little to teach patients," he noted.

The last category of education is in the area of human behavior. There is a need for behavioral science knowledge in the various specialties represented in the hospital, Mr. Connelly said, "and right now the educator has a great opportunity for providing that knowledge."

DISCUSSION

In response to a question about hospitals' affiliation with colleges and universities, Mr. Connelly agreed that this type of cooperative program would be another category of hospital education. A faculty member of a university hospital administration program expressed this idea about affiliation: "I think that we often fall into the trap of assuming that all education for persons who work in the hospital must take place in the hospital. We have seen it in the literature—the hospital is the cog of the community wheel, and it should reach out to all segments. Some of that is going to change, because if it does not, inefficiency can result. We need to ask, 'Can some of this education be accomplished more effectively outside hospital walls?' "

An adult educationist: What do you do for professional development for yourself and your staff?

Mr. Connelly: I have a staff of 19, 5 of whom are educators and the remainder of whom are professionals in other fields. We are doing our own training, teaching the noneducators educational theory and practice.

Adult educationist: What kind of career line is apparent to you in your own hospital?

Mr. Connelly: Nothing else. There is no upward mobility.

A university health administration faculty member: As the health field, especially the hospital, changes, educators like Walt will move up into corporate structures, being advisers to, say, a chief executive officer of a multiple hospital system. If educators do not assume the responsibility for educational administration in a hospital setting, an administrator— who may not know very much about education—will take over this advisory role at the top level. I hope that some educators will take the initiative for educational administration in hospitals.

In response to a question about whether growth in his staff had occurred at his request, Mr. Connelly replied: "In only two cases has it been at my request. In the others, it was imposed by administration."

A representative of a continuing education program in nursing: That worries me. It seems as though administration may be looking to education to solve some problems that can be solved only by other means. Our response in education frequently is not justified on the basis of research into what we can accomplish.

Mr. Connelly: There are instances in which education is used to substitute for management, but there is so much that education can accomplish in the hospital that the educator need not conduct programs to solve a management problem.

Nursing program representative: But are we attacking the problems with the wrong kinds of programs? I suspect that some of the educational programs that we conduct are inappropriate solutions to certain problems. If we contributed an equal amount of time, money, and personnel to solving some problems in other ways, then the problems might not even exist. For example, if the clinical practice of nursing were made more rewarding or if the position were restructured, nursing aides might not be needed and we could do away with nursing aide training. You see, I am not sure that a lot of our problems are educational problems.

Mr. Connelly: The education department must respond to the hospital's educational needs but must not push education for the sake of education.

An adult educationist: All morning we have talked about education in the hospital as though the activities of the training staff are the only activities that qualify as education. In your classification scheme, you included continuing education, but you did not comment on the extent to which what you do is antithetical to, complementary with, or isolated from what the directors of continuing medical education are trying to do.

Mr. Connelly: In our hospital, continuing medical education is totally separated from the kinds of activities that I am involved in. I suspect that this is true in most hospitals. (General agreement was expressed by the participants.)

Another adult educationist: I have heard you discussing the educational mission in terms of helping individuals to acquire new knowledge, skills, and capabilities. I have not heard much about the education department as a unit that helps other units to assess needs and to facilitate human development through a problem-solving and decision-making process in which those to be affected by the decisions will be involved in helping to formulate them. How do you handle that?

Mr. Connelly: In my view, the hospital field is so far away from that kind of approach that if someone with that point of view was employed, he would not last. Our staff works very hard to help persons to acquire those skills, but we have to do it informally. We are a long way from accomplishing what you are referring to.

Findings of a Functional Job Analysis

Patty Dunkel, research associate, HETP, summarized the findings of a functional job analysis of 587 members of the American Society for Health Manpower Education and Training. Her report on this study, which she conducted under the Hospitalwide Education and Training Project of the Hospital Research and Educational Trust, was distributed to participants prior to the conference and is included as Appendix B.

In describing the study, Ms. Dunkel said: "A functional job analysis questionnaire (Appendix C), which required respondents to indicate the frequency with which they performed 74 discrete tasks, was mailed to the 1,023 members of ASHET who might have been employed by provider institutions. Seven hundred and fifty-five, or 74 percent, of those surveyed returned questionnaires. The nonrespondents appear not to have severely biased the findings. The frequency with which the respondents performed the 74 tasks did not form a pattern. While it is possible that the frequency intervals used in the questionnaire were too broad or too narrow, it seems more likely that the lack of a pattern was related to the heterogeneity of the group.

"The 11 tasks considered by the respondents to be most important to success on the job fell into three categories: managing the education unit, providing educational services, and engaging in personal professional development. It was interesting that 49 percent ranked 'preparing a written plan of objectives' as important to success on the job but that only 22 percent believed that examining the work of the unit against this plan was important. Perhaps this indicates that written statements of objectives are perfunctory for education units or that changes in the institutional demands on the units occurred so rapidly that the written plans were outdated before they had been implemented. The objectives may have been written in such a manner that they did not aid in implementation. Perhaps achieving the written objectives was not as important as the method by which they were achieved, or perhaps the respondents were not held accountable for achieving their objectives.

"The tasks ranked 2 through 5 (see Table 14, Appendix B) suggest the respondents' attempts to secure agreement with and commitment to the services that they provided. This interpretation was supported by the fact that 'talking informally with department heads and administrators to determine the effectiveness of education and training' was the most frequently performed task in the educational evaluation grouping. The importance of securing agreement and commitment should not be surprising, because the answers to such questions as 'What should be taught?' 'To whom?' and 'How?' are necessarily value judgments. Success in providing educational services to employees of health care institutions depends on the responsiveness of the education staff to the variety of values held by various persons and groups within the institution."

DISCUSSION

Questions were raised about the statistic showing that 29 percent of the educators in health care institutions had listed high school diplomas as their highest academic credentials. Ms. Dunkel explained that the respondents who had not listed a degree or a nursing diploma or who were not designated as registered nurses on ASHET's membership list were counted as high school graduates. This category could include persons with a number of college credits but without a nursing diploma or a degree, she said.

An adult educationist: What is at stake is whether or not we assume that we are going to be dealing with persons having uniform entry qualifications for employment.

Ms. Dunkel: I think that you can assume that we are not. Among the respondents, there is not only a wide range in levels of academic achievement but also a wide variety in subject area concentration.

Adult educationist: But do we think that such diversity is good or bad? For instance, should the work group that will be dealing with degree programs consider preparatory degree programs, or should it assume that the profession of hospital education, which remains relatively flexible in terms of entry, provides some common experience after entry? It seems that there are enormous differences between these two assumptions.

Another adult educationist: I think that this is the kind of decision that should be made by the group working on degree programs. I think that these data are saying that there is a need for programs for both the bachelor's degree and the postbachelor's degree.

Adult educationist: I hope that we are not making some unquestioned assumptions about credentials.

Ms. Dunkel: Because there appears to be some confusion on the part of hospital administrators about what can be expected from the director of education and because administrators are accustomed to hiring persons with academic credentials, I think that it is likely that the credential will make a difference in terms of prestige.

Adult educationist: I acknowledge that there is a problem regarding what is accepted conventionally, but it seems to me that what we decide here and that what is done with the results of our efforts will affect the way in which credentials are used in hiring. We could conceivably reach a conclusion that said, in effect, "Don't hire anyone who has not been through that degree program." I hope that we do not, either advertently or inadvertently.

Ms. Dunkel: I hope that we do not. One of the reasons that we are asking you to include a behavioral component and a subject matter component in each curricular recommendation that you develop is to suggest that the degree is not as important as what the person can do. Because hospital directors of training are a heterogeneous group and probably will continue to be for a while, we have structured three different programs in which they can gain the necessary skills and competencies.

Adult educationist: Let me add to that by saying not only that it is likely that the heterogeneity will continue but also that we should plan to let it continue. (Agreement was expressed by most of the participants.)

A nursing educator: I have another concern regarding the diversity in academic background. Instead of the 11 tasks that emerged in this survey as the most important ones, totally different tasks might have emerged if the respondents' educational preparation had been different. I would be very concerned if we viewed our task to be the development of educational programs that would help directors of education to perform only these 11 tasks better.

Ms. Dunkel: I hope that we will not. This study is intended to serve as a supplement to the lectures and discussions of this morning, to your own experience, and to the paper on the findings of the HETP. I think that as curriculum planners you should consider the future work life of students, students' abilities and desires, and the best guesses of experts regarding the future of the profession. Certainly, your expertise and experience are necessary elements in the development of the curricular recommendations.

An adult educationist: I have a related concern. In the list of 74 job tasks, I could find no statements that are specific to health and hospitals, except those that say "help the institution to analyze this or that."

Another adult educationist: I watched for that, too, because it was interesting to see whether the list portrayed the environment.

A hospital administration program representative: If it is true that 29 percent of the directors of education do not have any kind of degree or diploma, this situation may be the basis for the current problems with hospital training. It is fine to talk about competency, but the approach of "Who are you? What is your union card?" cannot be overcome. The person without the credential just has no credibility in the hospital.

A director of training: I have been in my job for 10 years. Every time that I attempt to recruit an educator, I am amazed that I get applicants who are high school graduates, male, aged 35 to 40, and who have had eclectic teaching experience. They usually come with many recommendations on their teaching ability.

An adult educationist: Do you hire them?

Director of training: I do not hire them.

Nursing educator: Why not?

Director of training: Because they are in competition with applicants who have more advanced academic credentials and an experiential base that I find more suitable. That is not to say that these persons would not be successful, because their resumes and recommendations show that they have performed well in the past.

A university hospital administration faculty member: That is exactly the point that was being made—that the hospital environment is oriented toward credentials.

Director of training: That is right. At the gut level, my concern is for the credibility of my department. I cannot afford to hire the farm equipment salesman and to send him to housekeeping to assist with training. The first question that he will be asked is, "What is your background?" If he answers "I sold manure spreaders to farmers," my department has had it.

Findings of the Hospitalwide Education and Training Project

Robert J. Munk, research associate, HETP, summarized the findings of the HETP study of hospitalwide education and training functions that were implemented at 16 single hospital demonstration sites. A digest of these findings was distributed to participants prior to the conference; a complete report on the HETP, including the findings of a study of shared educational services at 17 hospital consortium sites, has been published in *Hospitalwide Education and Training* (Chicago: Hospital Research and Educational Trust, 1977), by Robert J. Munk and Marc Lovett.

Mr. Munk said: "Data were collected from documentary materials and from interviews that were conducted at the 16 single hospitals participating in the project. The demonstration sites had been selected so as to provide a variety of institutional sizes, types, and locales (urban, suburban, and rural).

"The HETP was designed to demonstrate the advantages and disadvantages of a variety of ways of structuring hospitalwide education and training programs. The most important criterion in assessing the structures of programs was found to be the degree of centralization of the overall hospital administration and of the hospitalwide education and training function.

"The advantages and disadvantages of various arrangements for education functions were found to depend on the congruity between the function and the hospital administration. That is, the most advantageous arrangement for a hospitalwide education function was the one that was most harmonious with the hospital administration in terms of degree of centralization. Centralized approaches to education and training were most effective in centralized settings; decentralized arrangements worked best in decentralized settings.

"In reviewing the list of categories of hospital education and training that were cited this morning, several questions can be asked: For what categories of personnel are we going to conduct preservice education? For what categories are we going to conduct inservice training? Upgrading of skills? Continuing education?"

It is not assumed, Mr. Munk said, that all hospital personnel will be involved in every kind of education, although there is a trend in that direction. "Education in hospitals probably started with inservice training for nursing personnel. Now it is spreading to many departments, and the new requirements of the Joint Commission on Accreditation for Hospitals reflect this trend. There will be an incredible amount of growth in community and patient education. So far, however, few training departments are doing this type of training," Mr. Munk said.

He described some hospital training directors as being part of the "cabinet" of the hospital administration, regularly providing information upon which top-level policy decisions are based. Other hospital directors of training may be called upon to run management development classes. The situations are vastly different, he said. "I am sure that this complicates the task of developing curriculums, but it is the situation that we encountered in the field during the course of this project."

"The question that we posed in undertaking this project was, 'How should a hospital organize a training function?' Our conclusion is that the administrator first must ask, 'What do I want this function to perform?' and 'How does that fit in with the overall patterns of decision making within this institution?' With the answers to these questions, the administrator can structure the hospital's educational activities. In a nutshell, the conclusion of the project is that the hospital should organize its education and training function so that it is consistent with the overall organization," Mr. Munk said.

This conclusion means that there is no single best structure for education and training, he pointed out, adding, "What that means for curriculum is that there may not be one best curriculum."

DISCUSSION

A director of training: Did you say that the administrator establishes the type of education or training department within a specific institution?

Mr. Munk: The conclusion of my report is that ideally he would. In reality, few administrators think about how to structure an education function. An administrator says, "I want a training director. I am not sure what I want him to do, but I need one."

A university hospital administration faculty member: Why should he structure it?

Mr. Munk: Some administrators may consciously decide not to structure an education function because they want this function to be highly responsive to changes within the institution. At the same time, a certain amount of structuring occurs whether planned for or not.

Hospital administration faculty member: I am not addressing that issue. If an administration brings in a competent person, why impose its ideas when that person knows more about the function than the administration does?

Mr. Munk: The competent person should not be brought in the door and just turned loose. His activities have to be supportive of ongoing activities, and from the outset, certain reporting relationships and certain working relationships must be established. This most basic level of structure has to be provided. It establishes whether one central unit should have charge of all educational activities or whether the training function should be decentralized and to what extent.

Hospital administration faculty member: The existence of a specific organizational policy that defines what education will be seems to depend very much on the administrator's feelings about education. A person who sees education as a vital component to the survival of the organization will have a policy.

Another university hospital administration faculty member: In your observations, did you find administrators themselves participating on a regular basis, for example, in teaching part of a management training course or a history of the institution? Did you find an institution that had inservice education as a regular part of daily activity?

Mr. Munk: Yes on both counts. In answer to your first question, there were some hospital administrators who regularly took an active part in some of the teaching programs within the institutions. They were about as rare as the one administrator who regularly attended—not sat in on but attended—classes that were being held. In answer to your second question, it is fairly common to find institutions in which inservice activities are scheduled regularly so that there would be one per week or per month.

A nursing educator: The study pointed out that the persons working in a decentralized setting probably had to be somewhat different from those in a centralized setting. Are we to assume that this conference will deal with a centralized education and training department? The presentations this morning seemed to be based on that point of view, and yet, there is a great movement toward decentralization. Are we talking about the preparation of personnel who will be dynamically involved in education and training functions in health care institutions, or are we talking about the preparation of a training director who will be involved only in issuing directives and in conferring with administrators? I think that there is a real difference, and I do not know where we are.

Ms. Dunkel: If you are talking about a master's degree program, you might assume that you are training an educator for a high-level position within the organization. Even then, he may or may not be consulted by administration about educational policy. He may or may not consult with department heads about implementation of policy. He may develop and teach courses only when he is asked. If you are talking about a preservice nondegree program, you might make other assumptions. These are decisions to be made by the work groups.

In summarizing the discussion, Ms. Dunkel said that the hospital "is not only a health care organization but also an educational institution. A great deal of education and training is being conducted in hospitals, but it is usually highly fragmented. The situations in which hospital directors of education will work are highly varied. Some will advise administration on educational policy and on solving organizational problems with education. Some will consult with department managers about training or departmental problems. Others will be told to develop a specific program such as orientation or supervisory training. Some will have a great deal of control over many resources, whereas others will have little formal control over only a few resources. Some will work in hospitals where administration has precise expectations for education and training, and others will have only general, perhaps unclear, mandates. There is a demand for training to help hospital directors of education to learn about the field and to prepare them to perform and to continue to perform effectively. This training may even help some of them to decide that the field is not for them."

Guidelines on Developing Curriculum

Leonard Nadler, professor, adult education and human resources development, School of Education, George Washington University, Washington, DC, the final speaker in the general session, outlined the possibilities that would be open to the work groups in developing recommendations on curriculum for the three educational programs. Mr. Nadler cited two major problems for participants in reaching their objective: a lack of solid data and a lack of agreement among them about what the job of an educator in the hospital is. "Nevertheless," he said, "given what we know now, what can we suggest in the way of learning outcomes that will enable the persons doing this job to do it better than they are doing it now?"

By the end of the conference, he said, these outcomes are to be in the form of a list for each of the three types of programs. "You might start the lists with a statement such as, 'By the end of this learning experience, the participant will be able to . . . .' Recognize that you are not going to produce statements that can withstand the attacks of all of your professional colleagues. Right now, however, the institutions sponsoring training programs do not have any recommendations," Mr. Nadler said.

The three sources from which to compile the lists, he continued, are (1) the findings of the two HETP studies, (2) the ideas and perspectives presented in the talks given today, and (3) the most important, your own experiences. "Each of you was selected because it was thought that you had something to offer that was unique and that should be heard. You are a heterogeneous group—purposely—because that is what this field is."

In further defining the tasks of the work groups, Mr. Nadler explained that three content areas—education, health and hospital systems, and administration or management—could be dealt with. "The degree program could be a bachelor's program, a master's program, or both. The preservice nondegree program should include the kinds of learning that would be helpful to someone new to the job. The inservice nondegree program should be for the person who already is working in the field but who believes that he needs to learn more."

Further distinctions were drawn between the inservice nondegree program and the degree program. The former, Mr. Nadler said, would not be concerned with meeting institutional requirements for degrees and probably would give the learner more options in choosing what to take. Also, an inservice program probably would be of shorter duration than a degree program.

Mr. Nadler placed one limitation on the development of the curricular recommendations: "Please do not get into how the skills will be taught, that is, through field experience, internships, courses, and so forth. How they will be taught is not necessary at this point. What is being asked for is, 'What should the learning be?' You might assume that some of the competencies that you recommend could be attained by reading, attending credit or noncredit courses, training on the job, or any number of other ways."

CURRICULAR RECOMMENDATIONS

Preservice Nondegree Program

Participants in the work group on curriculum for a preservice nondegree program were: H. Walton Connelly, leader; George F. Aker; James A. Brigham; Frank Malouff; Herman Mullins; Robert Shouldice; and George R. Wren. Patty L. Dunkel was recorder.

SUMMARY OF REPORT

H. Walton Connelly presented the report of the work group responsible for developing curricular recommendations for a preservice nondegree program for educators in health care institutions. A preservice nondegree program was defined by the group as a short-term training experience that could be conducted in a variety of settings, Mr. Connelly said. For example, some of the competencies could be developed by outside reading or by self-instructional packages to be completed at home. Some could be developed and refined through an intensive residential course conducted before, during, or after the home-study work. Because the person enrolling in this kind of program probably would have experience either in health care or in education but not in both, the group recommended that the student be allowed to demonstrate competency in his area of expertise and to select only those learning experiences that would develop competency in areas in which he demonstrated a weakness. It was assumed, Mr. Connelly said, that the person entering the program "would have good interpersonal skills and would already value education

21

as a way of solving organizational problems and of implementing policy." Mr. Connelly also pointed out that the program defines three broad areas of understanding: the hospital, management, and adult education.

RECOMMENDATIONS ON CURRICULUM

The curriculum for a preservice nondegree program for hospital educators should be designed to provide them with competencies in three broad areas. Upon completion of such a program, educators should be able to:

A. *Understand the hospital*
  1. Describe the hospital as a social system, including
     a. External pressures, such as those imposed by regulations, accreditation, licensure, community groups, and local government, and how they affect the education function
     b. Formal and informal power structures within the institution
     c. Role and function of the education department and its relationship to other organizational departments
  2. Seek opportunities for serving as an education advocate
  3. Describe the organizational determinants of human behavior in the hospital, including
     a. Relations among various categories of personnel as affected by their role perceptions and by the socialization inherent in their training
     b. The variety of educational requirements for entry into positions in the hospital
     c. The unique character of the learner's particular hospital, for example, the degree of centralization of decision making

B. *Understand hospital administration and management*
  1. Describe management functions and the concepts of one or more of the theories of organization held by authorities in the field
  2. Develop and use a departmental budget and program budgets
     a. Read and interpret departmental financial statements
     b. Determine and express cost-effectiveness in terms familiar to hospital administrators
     c. Understand and be able to prepare reports using elementary descriptive statistics
  3. Identify problems that may be solved by education, and suggest and test solutions

C. *Understand adult education*
  1. Describe and use an educational program planning process for individual, group, or mass education*
     a. Identify problems that can be solved by education
     b. Develop and refine program objectives
     c. Design a suitable program format, including
        (1) Resources — persons, facilities, materials
        (2) Leaders—those with the responsibility to guide, direct, question, and instruct
        (3) Methods, techniques, and devices to facilitate individual, group, and mass education
        (4) Time schedules indicating when the activity should occur and how long it should last
        (5) Sequence of events—arrangement of activities so that they will be maximally educative
        (6) Social reinforcement—management of the emotional aspects of interpersonal relations
        (7) Individualization—providing for individual learning differences
        (8) Clarification of roles and relations of learners, leaders, and resource persons
        (9) Criteria for evaluation
        (10) Clarification of design to such persons as participants, participants' supervisors, administrators, and leaders
     d. Fit format into hospital operations
        (1) Guide students into, through, and out of format
        (2) Finance the program
        (3) Modify hospital operations to allow time and resources for the program
        (4) Validate content
     e. Put plan into effect
     f. Measure and appraise results
  2. Describe the adult as a learner
     a. Factors that inhibit and facilitate learning
     b. Motivation to learn

---

*The program planning process used by this group was adapted from that presented by Cyril O. Houle in his *The Design of Education* (San Francisco: Jossey-Bass Inc., 1972).

    3. Apply program planning process to training others to train
    4. Demonstrate at least six different teaching behaviors
    5. Prepare a variety of educational materials such as workbooks and criterion tests
    6. Continue learning—that is, have the motivation and the skill to learn
       a. Describe and use available resources
       b. Develop a set of individual learning strategies

DISCUSSION

One of the adult educators suggested that the HETP might seek grant support for a qualified educational institution to prepare some of the self-instructional packages, which could then be loaned to hospitals that were hiring new persons as educators.

Another adult educator: How many employees in the student's hospital, other than the student's director, would have to be involved in making this program work, and who are they?

Mr. Connelly: We do not know who they are or how they will communicate with the director of education so that he can obtain the information that he needs about his hospital. That is a whole area that needs some serious exploration.

Adult educationist: Is there some way in which one can track down the stimuli in the environment of a newly appointed hospital educator to learn what questions he is asking, which might be quite different from the questions that we are answering? I'm talking about "the teachable moment."

Another adult educationist: At different stages of a person's work life, different needs surface. No one program can be designed that will meet all needs. The existence of a program might be just the facilitating mechanism. It might help the trainer to recognize or articulate a need.

A university health administration faculty member: There are data from other organizations. Trainers in industry are not a new phenomenon.

An adult educationist: Perhaps what we ought to be doing is collecting the data from industry to show that the use of educators is cost-effective.

ASHET representative: The educator also has to be convinced that he is cost-effective. How do you sell or promote this idea to an administrator if you cannot articulate the value of education in the hospital?

A university health administration faculty member: Hospital and health care administrators are educated in master's degree programs. I would be pleased to include in our curriculum a presentation explaining what the job of the educator is and what the training director can do for the administrator. The administrators who we now have are busy—it is difficult to reach them—but the students are impressionable. Get to the administrative residents. That is a long-term project, but I think that it will affect conditions in 25 years.

Another university health administration faculty member: We are doing that in the hospital administration program at Duke University, and the students are excited about this area. In fact, we now have two students who want to go into hospital education as a management career.

Inservice Nondegree Program

Participants in the work group on curriculum for an inservice nondegree program were: Barbara P. McCool, leader; Alan G. Cotzin; Howard W. Houser; Barbara Nichols; Donald Sanders; and Alan Thomas. Robert J. Munk was recorder.

SUMMARY OF REPORT

Barbara P. McCool, associate professor, department of health administration, Duke University, Durham, NC, reported on the recommendations of the group developing curriculum for an inservice nondegree program. This group, Ms. McCool explained, tried to design a program to meet the immediate needs of a director of education or of staff currently working in a hospital department of education.

Four major areas of competency were identified as being crucial to education and training staff in performing their functions effectively. The first area of competency, said Ms. McCool, is an understanding of and ability to apply the idea that the individual learner determines what he will learn and the behavior that he will modify. This assumption must be taken into account by education staff in planning and implementing training programs. Second, hospital educators must have an understanding of and an ability to assess the intended and unintended consequences of training programs. The third area of competency is an understanding of the hospital environment, and the fourth, an ability to serve as an advocate for education within that environment.

Ms. McCool cautioned that the recommended competencies could not be attained by attending one short course of several days' duration. Depending on the background of the learner, she said, these competencies might be developed by outside reading and by study at home, plus participation in residential short courses and/or college or university noncredit courses.

RECOMMENDATIONS ON CURRICULUM

Upon completion of an inservice nondegree program, hospital educators should be able to design educational programs for hospital employees that demonstrate their understanding of:

A. *The learner as an individual,* including, but not limited to
   1. Individual learning styles
   2. Entry behaviors
   3. Social constraints to adult participation in learning activities
   4. Reinforcements to and constraints on applying new knowledge on the job
B. *Methods of assessing the intended and unintended consequences of an educational program,* including, but not limited to
   1. Establishing evaluation criteria
   2. Applying methods of collecting and analyzing data
   3. Making judgments from data that have been analyzed
   4. Explaining the costs incurred in developing and implementing an educational program
   5. Developing and using an educational information system
C. *The hospital environment,* including
   1. Constraints on the training function, such as lack of access to administration and effects of socialization among representatives of the various disciplines within the hospital
   2. Changes in authority and dependency relations between patient and physician, teacher and student, professional and client
   3. Implications for education of current issues in health care
D. *The need for the educator to serve as an advocate of education in the hospital,* including the ability to convince hospital personnel at various levels of their responsibility for their own continued learning and for that of their staff members

Degree Program

Participants in the work group on curriculum for a degree program were: William S. Griffith, leader; John C. Booth; Margaret E. Courtney; David R. Day; Nancy Diekelmann; Rose Kennedy; Barbara Knudson; Leonard Nadler; and Coolie Verner. Jeffrey Butler was recorder.

SUMMARY OF REPORT

This work group was unanimous in agreeing that education is the core of the training of a hospital director of education. In presenting the group's curricular recommendations for a degree program, William S. Griffith, associate professor and chairman, Committee on Educational Design and Implementation, Department of Education, University of Chicago, said: "Training in education is not something that is ancillary to administrative or sociological insights and skills and other leadership capabilities. Accordingly, we focused most heavily on the need to develop competent adult educators who would work in a hospital setting. Our assumption was that the adult educators are likely to have had prior practical management experience in some type of organization."

Two members of the group, however, hoped that the group's recommendations would not arbitrarily restrict the entrance of persons who lacked practical experience, Mr. Griffith said. "This was clearly a minority viewpoint," he added.

"We began by trying to spell out a few of the competencies that the educator working in the hospital setting ought to have. We tried to hit upon some of those that were most often overlooked in the practice of education in hospitals," he pointed out.

The group strongly believed, Mr. Griffith emphasized, that "at no point should we think of developing a profession that is a stepping stone to something else. The competencies identified certainly should not be regarded as an exhaustive list. In designing a degree program, the educationist ought to draw upon the extensive literature of competencies of adult educators and upon the strength that already exists in over 150 graduate programs in adult education in the United States.

"In addition, the programs now being conducted for hospital administrators ought to be regarded as providing potential components to be used in framing specific degree programs for directors of hospital education and training," Mr. Griffith said.

RECOMMENDATIONS ON CURRICULUM

A. *Competencies in education.* Adult educators who are being prepared to work as directors of hospital education and training should be able to:
   1. Assess learning needs by comparing competencies with required behaviors
   2. Determine whether prerequisite learning has been accomplished
   3. Write instructional objectives
   4. Identify and specify the learning tasks involved in achieving each objective
   5. Select and use instructional materials and equipment appropriate for achieving specific objectives
   6. Select and use instructional techniques appropriate for achieving specific objectives
   7. Understand and apply principles of adult learning
   8. Evaluate the effectiveness of an educational program
   9. Manage the learning environment

B. *Competencies in understanding the hospital as a social system.* Directors of education and training in hospitals should be able to:
   1. Understand and use, *as appropriate*, the traditional educational practice associated with each professional and occupational group within the hospital
   2. Establish a learning environment appropriate to each of the different groups of learners in the hospital
   3. Understand the prerogatives and territoriality of the various professional and occupational groups
   4. Understand the management processes in hospitals, for example, the unique role of the hospital administrator
   5. Identify the unique constraints imposed by licensure, certification, and other types of legal requirements on defining permissible job functions in the hospital
   6. Understand the distinctive role of the hospital in dealing with morbidity and mortality
   7. Appreciate the fact that the learners in a hospital believe that their situation is unique
   8. Understand the limitations imposed by the divided authority that exists in the hospital setting, in particular, the relative independence of physicians

9. Understand the unique influences imposed by external organizations on hospitals, including regulatory requirements, financial restrictions, and professional requirements
10. Understand the effects that changes in the health care system have had, are having, and will have on education in the hospital
11. Be aware of the implications of multiple short career ladders in hospitals, such as limited upward mobility
12. Be conversant with the various technical vocabularies used in the hospital

C. *Competencies in education management.* Directors of education in hospitals should be able to:
1. Understand the constraints imposed by cost reimbursement practices on educational programming
2. Understand the implications of cost-benefit concepts for educational programming
3. Be able to reconcile the possible conflict between the urge to provide learning for all adults in the hospital and the restrictions imposed by organizational goals and limited resources
4. Understand the effects that manpower planning might have on future educational programming

DISCUSSION

A representative of a university health administration program: Is this an implied master's degree program?

Mr. Griffith: We were talking about either a baccalaureate or a master's degree program, but in every case, the program would be for persons with practical backgrounds. Graduate education would suggest greater depth, in knowledge of a more theoretical nature.

An adult educationist: Most adult educators work alone, and they work on the learner's ground. This is a situation entirely different from what most other educators face. Could one include in a curriculum, in addition to the importance of understanding the hospital, some reflection of the implications of adult education in other noneducational institutions?

Mr. Griffith: That is part of what we are saying in one of our recommendations—that educators should be able to manage their learning environments.

Adult educationist: Also, we should be responsible for describing the historical context in which we are developing these recommendations. In five years, the role of director of education in hospitals no longer will be novel. The directors now are fighting an entirely new battle. There are all kinds of difficulties, but there also is excitement.

Another adult educationist: It is not brand new. It has been going on for 20 years. We should try to capture what has been going on in those 20 years to show that there is a history. What is different is that more attention is being paid to it than before. Maybe an understanding of why will indicate where some of the emphasis should be.

Hospital administration faculty member: In these outlines of the three programs, we have created three good job descriptions.

ASHET representative: The emphasis has to be on the function, and the job description will result from that. What we have never had is a clear definition of the function. Depending on the size of the hospital, the resources available, and the overall organizational structure, the job description will fall into place. In 1970, the U.S. Department of Labor issued a job description, but it does not touch on much of what is in these reports.

Another hospital administration faculty member: If you are talking about a standardized job description, I am not sure that one is desirable, given the variety of settings that we are talking about.

Mr. Griffith: One would have to keep in mind that those who theorize about curriculum development draw their notions about objectives from a variety of sources. One of these sources is what is currently going on in the field. Another source is the set of predictions of scholars in the field of what is likely to happen. A third source is a sense of values: "What is it that we *should* be doing?" A fourth is "What do the potential students think that they want to learn?" If a curriculum developer overlooked any one of these sources, he might get into serious trouble in designing a program. It is likely that he also would be in trouble if he focused exclusively on any one of these sources.

An adult educationist: Most of the emphasis in the degree program seems to be on the individual learner's acquiring competencies to enable him to perform his job more effectively. The role of education and training for groups of persons collectively learning to achieve organizational goals could fit into the scheme but seems not to be highlighted anywhere.

A director of training: The general perspective in the hospital is that the educator gets involved only at an individual level, albeit the individual may be in a group. The technique of working with a group to enable it to become more effective, which sometimes is referred to as organizational development, has been notoriously unsuccessful in hospitals. We certainly need to be looking in that direction.

SUMMARY

A vast amount of education is being conducted in health care institutions. Eleven types of programs, ranging from preservice training for employees to health education for patients and members of the community, were cited by the participants of this conference as falling within the scope of education in the hospital. In most instances, medical education and continuing medical education are not the responsibility of educators in health care institutions, and the extent to which the other types are varies considerably from one institution to another. Whether the hospital is the only, or, indeed, the proper, place in which to conduct these programs is a question that administrators are beginning to raise and would like to see addressed. In developing their recommendations for curriculums for hospital educators, the participants acknowledged the need for applying some degree of coordination and control to educational programming in the hospital.

Heterogeneity—of the occupational group, of the conditions under which its members work, and of the group of participants itself—was a recurring theme throughout the conference. It generally was agreed that this heterogeneity is appropriate to the present condition of health care institutions and that educational programs directed toward persons working as or wishing to become educators in these institutions should be based on the assumption that heterogeneity is appropriate. It also was agreed that, because of this situation, there could be no one "best" curriculum for this group of educators.

Despite the heterogeneity of the group, there were some conditions and problems that appeared to be common to all educators in health care institutions. Limited career mobility was cited as a current major problem. Participants also identified several problems inherent in establishing a new role in an existing social system. One of these was the uncertainty of administrators regarding the skills that an educator should be expected to have. Also emerging from the discussions was uncertainty about the structure of the job of the educator and about what should be expected, in terms of performance, of the person holding the position. The participants generally agreed that, although the uncertainties inherent in establishing a new role in an existing system would continue to exist for a while, they would be subject to modification over time. However, they emphasized that, until such change occurred, the uncertainties would have vast implications for the training of persons to fill the position.

Another condition that was cited as common to educators in health care institutions is that they work alone, or with a relatively small group of other persons, on the learner's ground and thus are unlike educators in public and private schools because they face a different set of constraints upon their activities and a different set of socializing influences. It was agreed that this difference has vast implications for curriculum development.

Participants expressed concern about the effect that their recommendations might have on the credential system in the health care institution. They acknowledged that a credential is important for the educator to have in establishing credibility with hospital administration but that it is lowly correlated with ability. They could not agree on recommending a specific credential that should be required for hospital educators.

The participants did agree on two basic recommendations. The first is that curriculums for hospital educators should be designed not only to increase educators' skill in conducting current activities but, more importantly, to enable them to develop new ways of performing their jobs and to assist hospital administrators in making more profitable use of their skills. The second recommendation is that existing programs of adult education or hospital administration be utilized as a basis for developing curriculums for educators in health care institutions.

Recommendations on Future Activities

The presentations and discussions of the conference give rise to ideas for future activities that will help to prepare educators in health care institutions for their unique role and responsibilities. These activities are as follows:

- Preparation of a learning package that could be used in hospital administration courses or by administrators in hospitals to describe the wide variety of possible roles and functions of a hospital educator, the skills required of the persons who assume these roles, and some of the limitations inherent in the roles.

- Preparation of a learning package on the hospital as a social system that could be used not only by educators but also by other professionals new to the health care institution.

- Preparation of learning packages based on any subset of the curricular recommendations developed by conference participants.

- Development of a preservice nondegree program for educators who have experience in other fields but who are new to the health care field.

- Development of a preservice nondegree program for health care personnel who are assuming educational responsibilities for the first time. This program and the one suggested for educators with experience in other fields could be developed and administered by any of the organizations or by any combination of the organizations represented at the conference.

- Securing of tuition for persons already working as educators in health care institutions, to enable them to enroll in a degree program designed around the recommendations of this conference and conducted in such a way that students could continue working.

- Development and conducting of programs to explore further some of the problems identified during the conference. Such programs could focus on the questions that educators in health care institutions are asking at various stages of their careers, on the history of education in health care institutions, and on the reasons for the current interest in the differentiation of the education function.

Closing Remarks

In closing the conference on behalf of the Hospital Research and Educational Trust, Herbert K. Gatzke said to the participants: "You have provided us with several things. One is an excellent base for our own further planning and action. I am convinced that the various disciplines represented here indeed can work together to help improve the quality of programs carried on in hospitals. Your discussions and recommendations have an air of reality about them. We thank you for that and for your interest, your time, and your contributions."

Appendix A

Glossary

Competency statement	A description of the skills, knowledge, or sensitivities characteristic of the persons holding a particular position or doing the work toward which an educational program is directed. A competency statement normally includes two elements: a description of expected student behavior and a description of the subject matter or content to which the behavior applies.
Degree program	A sequence of learning experiences intended to assist persons in increasing their skills, knowledge, or sensitivities, leading to an associate, baccalaureate, master's, or doctoral degree.
Educationist	One who studies the process of education.
Educator	A person who assists others in improving themselves or their society by increasing their skills, knowledge, or sensitivities in a particular subject area.
Expertise	A high degree of skill, knowledge, or sensitivity in a certain subject area. Expertise may be achieved through a systematic educational pro-

cess, through the assimilation of life experience, or through both.

Inservice nondegree program

A sequence of learning experiences intended to assist persons already engaged in an occupation in increasing their skills, knowledge, or sensitivities. No degree is conferred upon completion of the program.

Preservice nondegree program

A sequence of learning experiences intended to assist persons in increasing their skills, knowledge, or sensitivities, as preparation for a specific occupation. No degree is conferred upon completion of the program.

Appendix B

A Functional Job Analysis of Educators in Health Care Institutions: Implications for Higher and Continuing Education Curriculums

by
Patty L. Dunkel

Introduction

The late 1950s and the early 1960s witnessed an increased interest on the part of health care institutions in the continuing education and training of health manpower. The nine-year Hospital Continuing Education Project was funded, beginning in 1964, by a grant from the W. K. Kellogg Foundation, Battle Creek, MI, to the Hospital Research and Educational Trust, an affiliate of the American Hospital Association (AHA). Its objective was to establish a network for communication and cooperation among health manpower educators and trainers[1] and to promote the concept of hospitalwide education and training. In 1972, the Hospitalwide Education and Training Project (HETP) was funded through a grant from the Kellogg Foundation to the Trust. Its primary purpose was to demonstrate a variety of organizational models for education and training in health care institutions through the study of 33 demonstration sites that were or that proposed to be actively involved in the provision of hospitalwide education and training. A second objective of the project was to develop recommendations for preservice and continuing education curriculums for persons who were or who planned to become educators and trainers in health care institutions.

This report describes a study that was conducted under the HETP to help meet the second objective. It presents the findings of a functional job analysis of the occupation "educator/trainer" in health care institutions, which was designed to be used by curriculum planners in higher and continuing education. In addition to presenting the significant activities of hospital educators, the report explains the rationale for the study, the method of data collection, and the implications that the findings have for curriculums.

Rationale for the Study

Ultimately, curricular decisions are conscious choices, value judgments made by those responsible for an educational program. How are these decisions made? Are they based only on the personal preferences of individuals or of groups? Although the philosophy of the decision makers can significantly influence their curricular choices, certain types of information will provide them with a more intelligent basis for applying their philosophies to the decision-making process.[2]

There are three fundamental sources of information that aid in making curricular decisions: the nature of the subject matter, the characteristics of the students, and the conditions of contemporary life.[3] Information derived from the nature of subject matter usually is obtained by asking subject specialists what their subject can contribute to the education of persons who are not going to be specialists in that field. Studies of the students in an educational program would attempt to identify their interests and capacities and to determine needed changes in their behavior patterns.* Studies of contemporary life usually examine some manageable phase of life, such as societal expectations of the health care delivery system and the implications of those expectations for health care institutions. Frequently, studies of contemporary life for occupational curriculums focus on the activities of the practitioner or on the conditions under which the activities are performed.[4]

---

*In this report, "behavior patterns" refer to thinking and feeling as well as to overt actions.

Data from the first two sources are readily available to persons responsible for curricular decisions, but data from the third source are not. Although the literature regarding hospital education and training contains descriptions of specific programs, materials, and services, there is little explicit information about the process of developing these products.

On the assumption that preservice and continuing education curriculums should be directed in part toward preparing the employee to perform his job, the HETP staff decided that a detailed description of what the hospital educator does in the course of his work would be useful to curriculum developers.

When the curriculum aspect of the HETP was designed, staff doubted that the 33 project directors adequately represented the universe of educators in health care institutions. Thus, it was decided that a larger number of educators and trainers in health care institutions should be surveyed and that members of the American Society for Health Manpower Education and Training (ASHET), a personal membership organization of the AHA, would be an excellent source from which to obtain information.

There are at least two well-established techniques for systematically obtaining data on activities performed by an occupational group: critical incident analysis and functional job analysis. Critical incident analysis requires gathering information and writing detailed descriptions of events judged to be fundamental to a positive or negative occupational rating.[5] Functional job analysis is the process of determining the significant activities or tasks that constitute a specific job by observing the worker perform the job or by questioning the worker about the job.[6] Inferences about the necessary cognitive skills and the content to which the skills are applied are made from an examination of the data collected by either technique.

The collection of a large number of critical incidents, written in the specified format, presented staff with the following problems:

- How to select the writers to ensure that the great variety of institutional settings in which trainers work would be adequately represented
- How to train the writers in the critical incident process
- How to compensate the writers
- What framework to use in analyzing the incidents

Functional job analysis, on the other hand, had been used to collect data from which curricular objectives for a number of occupational groups had been derived, including librarians,[7] health care workers,[8] and police personnel.[9] For the study of each of these three occupations, data were obtained from a large number of workers by questionnaire. It was decided that this technique would be the more effective one to use in collecting data for curriculum development.

Data Collection

DEVELOPMENT OF QUESTIONNAIRE

A task analysis questionnaire (Appendix C) was developed to assess the frequency with which educators and trainers in health care institutions performed 74 discrete tasks.* The development involved three stages: first, the range and variety of tasks performed by persons involved in health manpower education and training were established through a review of the literature, an analysis of the reports of the 33 project directors, and interviews with six educators from health care institutions; second, a list of statements of discrete tasks was prepared; and third, a pilot study was conducted to test the comprehensibility of the questionnaire.

Articles about education in health care institutions were collected from the 1974 and 1975 issues of *Cross-Reference,* a newsletter published by the AHA for persons involved in hospital education and training, and *Hospitals, Journal of the American Hospital Association.* Based on an analysis of these articles, 120 discrete task statements were compiled. The analysis of the project directors' reports revealed an additional 95 tasks.

Three hundred specific task statements were developed from interviews that were conducted with six educators in health care institutions. To encourage the educators to think about the questions before the interview, letters were mailed describing the purpose of the study and specifying the questions to be discussed. The educators interviewed were:

- The director of hospitalwide education and training for a 650-bed teaching hospital, which also was affiliated with a vocational-

---

*Although 72 numbered task statements appear on the questionnaire, one is a three-part statement requiring three discrete responses.

technical school. The director had a master's degree in guidance and counseling and had been employed in the department for six years. During the past three years, he had been director. The department was approximately eight years old.

• The director of hospital education for a 112-bed community hospital that was not affiliated with any educational institutions. The director was completing a program leading to a master's degree in public health and had held his position for approximately one year. The department was approximately five years old.

• The director of education for a 511-bed, church-operated hospital that offered degree and certificate programs through a four-year college. The director had a bachelor's degree in business and had held his position for approximately three years. The department was approximately five years old.

• The director of nursing inservice education for a 200-bed community hospital, which conducted licensed practical nurse and nursing aide training in cooperation with a city school system. The director also was responsible for some interdepartmental training. The director was a graduate of a diploma school of nursing and had held this position for 11 years.

• The director of education and training for a three-hospital system with a total of 878 beds. The system conducted educational programs in cooperation with a city school system. The director had a master's degree in education and was the first person to hold this position, which had been in existence for approximately three years.

• A staff member of the department of education in a 405-bed community hospital. The staff member was a former secondary school teacher and had held the hospital position for approximately two years.

Before starting each interview, the interviewer made certain that the participant understood the purpose and process of the interview. The first question asked was: "What do you consider to be the three or four most important things that you do as (title of educator)?" After the participant stated three or four activities, the interviewer then asked: "How do you conduct (the activity cited)?" or "What do you do when you (the activity cited)?" The interviews were conducted in a manner to encourage maximum response from the educators. Each interview lasted approximately one to one and one-half hours.

Tapes and notes were transcribed on the same day that the interview was conducted. To ensure reliability, the interviewer and another staff member each analyzed the information recorded and compiled a list of task statements. The two lists agreed 100 percent.

Because the task statements appeared to contain many duplications, staff determined whether the same task was covered in more than one statement. This process reduced the number of statements to 71. The statements were edited by a staff member of the AHA's Division of Research and then incorporated in a questionnaire.

The questionnaire asked respondents to identify the organization in which they were employed as a health care institution, a consortium of health care institutions, or another type of organization. It also asked for pertinent information about the organization and about the background and current position of the respondent. The respondents then were asked to indicate the number of times during the past year that they personally had performed each of the 71 tasks listed. Finally, they were asked to select from the 71 tasks five or fewer that they considered most important to success in their job.

To pretest the questionnaire, copies were mailed to the directors of projects at 31 of the HETP demonstration sites. Twenty-nine questionnaires were returned. Of the two not returned, one was from a consortium that temporarily was without a director and one was from a single hospital. In addition to responding to the questionnaire, the project directors were asked to indicate any tasks that they performed that had been omitted from the list. Those who listed additional tasks or made other comments were interviewed by telephone to verify the correct wording of the task statements.

As a result of the pretest, three task statements were added to the questionnaire, and the section on frequency of performance was revised. This revision was necessary because some of the tasks were not performed routinely and could not be incorporated in the response categories. The final questionnaire is included in Appendix C.

DISTRIBUTION AND SORTING OF QUESTIONNAIRES

Because some of the members of the American Society for Health Manpower Education and Training were not affiliated with health care providers, the ASHET membership list was examined, and the names of persons for whom the questionnaire was not intended were deleted. Questionnaires were mailed to 1,023 members on March 8, 1976. A follow-up mailing was made on March 25 to those who had not responded to the first mailing. The two mailings resulted in the receipt of 696 responses. To increase the response rate, all nonrespondents for whom business addresses were available and whose titles suggested that they might be involved in hospital education were telephoned and urged to complete and return the questionnaire. This effort resulted in the receipt of 59 additional questionnaires, a total of 755, or 74 percent.

Of the 268 nonrespondents, 26 were employed by organizations whose names suggested that they were not provider institutions but possibly lead agencies in consortiums. Ten of the 26 nonrespondents were selected randomly and telephoned; none was involved in a consortium.

Another 82 nonrespondents had titles of "assistant administrator," "director of personnel," or "assistant director of nursing." Twenty of these persons were selected randomly and telephoned; none was responsible for education and training. Of the 40 whose titles suggested involvement with training, 18 were no longer in their jobs, and their replacements had not been selected. The remaining 22 did not form a pattern in terms of geography, length of membership, or size of institution. The only information available for the remaining 120 nonrespondents was home address and year of affiliation with ASHET. Geographic or length-of-membership patterns could not be discerned for this group.

Of the 755 ASHET members who responded to the questionnaire, 42 were employed by consortiums. Because it seemed unlikely that institutions of higher or continuing education would be interested in developing curriculums for the small number of persons employed by consortiums, these responses were not included in the analysis. Eighty-nine responses from ASHET members who were employed by organizations other than health care institutions or consortiums also were excluded.

Six hundred and twenty-four of the respondents, or approximately 83 percent, were employed by provider institutions. Thirty-eight responses from educators in health care institutions were excluded from the analysis. Eight of these were returned with the notation that the persons to whom they were addressed were no longer there; 25 respondents failed to complete one or more pages and thus did not give an accurate picture of their activities; and 5 spent less than 50 percent of their time in educational activities. Thus, responses from a total of 587 educators in health care institutions were used as the basis for analysis.

Findings

When this study was planned, it was hypothesized that the variables represented by the questions regarding institutional and personal characteristics could make a significant difference in the activity pattern of the educator and that, consequently, an analysis of variance technique would be needed to establish differences in activity patterns. However, a preliminary analysis of the data revealed little difference in frequency of performance or of perceived importance, based on any of these variables. It is true that educators who did not have a nursing background did not teach nursing subjects or analyze patients' records to determine training activities. It also is true that the frequency of attending committee meetings, of assisting the administrative staff in planning decision-making meetings, and of conducting or serving as a mediator in such meetings was related to length of time in the position. However, the overall activity pattern did not vary meaningfully with any of the hypothesized variables. Thus the data will be presented in aggregate form.

FREQUENCY OF PERFORMANCE OF TASKS

Planning and Organizing Departmental Work

The frequency with which educators in health care institutions performed four tasks related to planning and organizing the work of the education unit is shown in Table 1. The following were the most common responses: 48 percent of the respondents prepared a written plan of objectives and priorities once or twice a year; 43 percent examined the work of the unit in light of the established plan from 3 to 12 times per year; 40 percent reviewed changes in institutional policies to determine the effect of such changes on the unit from 3 to 12 times per year; and 34 percent found it necessary to adjust the assignments of their personnel 12 or fewer times per year.

Managing and Developing Staff

Table 2 displays the frequency with which educators in health care institutions performed 11 tasks regarding management and staff development. Although no clear frequency pattern emerges from this grouping, the majority of respondents performed each task during the past year, whether they were managers or staff members of the unit.

Budgeting

Table 3 shows the frequency of performance of budgeting tasks. Sixty-nine percent of the respondents said that budgets were prepared and submitted to administration once or twice during the past year; 44 percent said that the assigned budget was allocated once or twice per year; and 11 percent said that it was allocated from 3 to 12 times per year. Forty percent of the educators did not report expenditures to administration, possibly because this task was done by computer or because the education budget was not sufficient to warrant routine reporting.

TABLE 1. *Percent of Educators Who Performed Departmental Planning and Organizing Tasks, by Frequency of Performance*

	Frequency (N=587)						
Task	0 times	1-2 times	3-12 times	13-50 times	51-100 times	100 or more times	No answer
1. Prepared a written plan of objectives and priorities for education and training unit	5	48	32	12	3	–	–
2. Examined the work of education and training unit in light of established objectives and priorities	4	26	43	19	6	1	1
3. Reviewed changes in hospital policies and procedures to determine effect on education and training unit	9	23	40	21	4	3	–
4. Adjusted the assignment of education and training personnel to meet work demands	18	14	34	23	5	5	1

TABLE 2. *Percent of Educators Who Performed Education Staff Development Tasks, by Frequency of Performance*

Task	0 times	1-2 times	3-12 times	13-50 times	51-100 times	100 or more times	No answer
				Frequency (N=587)			
1. Informed education and training staff of policy or procedural changes that affect their work	15	10	31	30	8	5	1
2. Conducted education and training unit staff meetings to coordinate activities	21	8	31	31	7	1	1
3. Reviewed program designs and reports prepared by education and training personnel	17	13	33	27	6	3	1
4. Conducted inservice training for education and training personnel	31	17	35	12	2	2	1
5. Resolved differences among education and training employees	40	26	24	8	–	1	1
6. Interviewed prospective education and training personnel	43	25	26	5	–	–	1
7. Selected prospective education and training personnel	48	34	17	–	–	–	1
8. Developed job descriptions for education and training personnel	24	52	22	1	–	–	1
9. Set performance standards for education and training personnel based on organizational priorities	32	35	26	5	1	–	1

(continued on next page)

TABLE 2. *(continued)*

Task	0 times	1-2 times	3-12 times	13-50 times	51-100 times	100 or more times	No answer
			Frequency (N=587)				
10. Conducted perform-ance appraisals of education and train-ing personnel based on personal knowl-edge and data rele-vant to job perform-ance	28	34	32	4	1	–	1
11. Made recommenda-tions for promotions, transfers, and salary increases for educa-tion and training personnel	36	33	26	4	–	–	1

TABLE 3. *Percent of Educators Who Performed Budgeting Tasks,
by Frequency of Performance*

Task	0 times	1-2 times	3-12 times	13-50 times	51-100 times	100 or more times	No answer
			Frequency (N=587)				
1. Prepared suggested budgets covering edu-cation and training operations for submis-sion to administration	21	69	9	1	–	–	–
2. Allocated the budget assigned to education and training	36	44	11	4	1	2	2
3. Reported to adminis-tration expenditures to date	40	31	24	4	–	–	1

Other Administrative Tasks

Educators in health care institutions spent time performing other administrative tasks, as Table 4 indicates. Forty-one percent prepared written reports for administration about the education of the institution's personnel from 3 to 12 times per year. Fifty-four percent developed a system for recording data about the education of these personnel once or twice during the year.

Participation in Interdepartmental Activities

The frequency with which educators participated in interdepartmental activities that might not be considered strictly educational is shown in Table 5. The majority performed four of these six tasks; regarding the other two tasks, only 33 percent mediated disagreements among managers of other organizational units, and only 40 percent served on committees to establish organizational budget priorities.

TABLE 4. *Percent of Educators Who Performed Administrative Tasks, by Frequency of Performance*

Task	0 times	1-2 times	3-12 times	13-50 times	51-100 times	100 or more times	No answer
1. Prepared written reports for administration and/or other managers about the education and training of employees	10	26	41	19	2	1	1
2. Developed a system for recording data about the education and training of employees of the organization	21	54	20	3	–	1	1
3. Maintained such a system	24	35	15	10	3	10	3
4. Initiated or responded to correspondence regarding education and training procedures, activities, and services	2	8	42	35	7	6	–
5. Typed correspondence	62	11	10	9	3	4	1

Frequency (N=587)

TABLE 5. *Percent of Educators Who Performed Interdepartmental Tasks Not Considered Strictly Educational, by Frequency of Performance*

Task	Frequency (N=587)						
	0 times	1-2 times	3-12 times	13-50 times	51-100 times	100 or more times	No answer
1. Assisted others in setting up new systems, writing procedure manuals, and the like	15	28	41	13	2	1	–
2. Served as a member of hospital committees to:							
a. Review various hospital policies	21	19	35	17	3	1	4
b. Establish hospital budget priorities	48	21	14	4	1	–	12
c. Resolve specific hospital problems	15	20	40	15	3	2	5
3. Suggested ways, other than education and training, for dealing with organizational problems	9	26	47	15	3	–	–
4. Assisted the administrative staff in planning decision-making meetings	39	21	26	10	2	1	1
5. Conducted or served as a mediator in decision-making meetings	47	20	22	8	2	1	–
6. Mediated disagreements among managers of other organizational units	66	15	14	3	1	–	1

Assessing Training Needs

Table 6 shows the frequency with which 12 methods of assessing institutional training needs were performed. Fifty-one percent of the respondents developed education and training activities and/or services at the request of department heads or administration from 3 to 12 times during the past year; 50 percent analyzed current hospital problems to determine the need for new or changed programs with the same frequency. Forty percent conducted carefully planned interviews from 3 to 12 times per year, and 40 percent talked informally with department heads 13 to 50 times. Ninety-five percent or more of the educators spent some time during the past year assessing educational needs by talking informally with department heads, analyzing current institutional problems, and responding to requests from department managers or administration. This finding agrees with Schechter's finding that interviews with supervisors, department heads, and administrative staff, together with informal conversation, were the methods most frequently used to determine training needs.[10]

Providing Educational Services and Materials

The respondents indicated that they provided a variety of educational services and materials from 3 to 12 times during the past year, as shown in Table 7. Fifty-seven percent recommended training to resolve specific performance problems, and 52 percent evaluated machinery or equipment and recommended purchase. All tasks in this category were performed from 3 to 12 times per year, except planning and developing individualized instructional programs. Forty-six percent of the respondents did not perform this task, although 75 percent assisted others in performing it.

Teaching

Educators in health care institutions commonly teach courses in a variety of subject areas, as shown in Table 8. Ninety-six percent of the respondents taught some courses; 30 percent taught from 3 to 12 times during the past year, and 28 percent, from 13 to 50 times. Of the 561 who taught, 59 percent, all of whom had nursing backgrounds, taught nursing subjects, and 51 percent, who had widely varying backgrounds, taught management and supervisory development. That the respondents did not teach certain subjects does not mean that those subjects were not taught by someone else in the institution.

TABLE 6. *Percent of Educators Who Performed Needs Analysis Tasks, by Frequency of Performance*

Task	Frequency (N=587)						
	0 times	1-2 times	3-12 times	13-50 times	51-100 times	100 or more times	No answer
1. Talked informally with department heads and administrative staff to determine possible education and training activities	2	8	35	40	10	5	–
2. Conducted carefully planned interviews with department heads, administrative staff, and other personnel to determine possible education and training activities	18	21	40	17	3	1	–
3. Prepared and distributed questionnaires to learn about possible education and training activities	24	36	35	4	–	1	–
4. Analyzed the job descriptions of various hospital staff to ascertain possible education and training activities	31	29	34	6	–	–	–
5. Analyzed existing organizational policies to determine possible education and training activities	20	34	37	8	1	–	–
6. Analyzed hospital or departmental procedure manuals to determine possible education and training activities	23	30	35	10	1	1	–

(continued on next page)

TABLE 6. (continued)

Task	0 times	1-2 times	3-12 times	13-50 times	51-100 times	100 or more times	No answer
7. Analyzed current hospital problems or interests to determine the need for new training and education programs or changes in existing programs	5	15	50	24	4	2	—
8. Analyzed patients' records in light of staff capabilities to determine education and training activities	44	14	24	13	3	1	1
9. Planned or assisted others in planning task analysis studies to specify skills and knowledge required for various positions	39	28	26	6	1	—	—
10. Observed the work of personnel in other organizational units to help determine problems amenable to training	36	25	30	7	1	1	—
11. Assisted in the specification of competencies or criteria for various jobs in the hospital	43	27	25	4	1	—	—
12. Developed training and education activities and/or services in response to requests from department heads or administrative staff	5	14	51	24	3	3	—

Frequency (N=587)

TABLE 7. *Percent of Educators Who Performed Tasks Regarding Provision of Educational Materials and Services, by Frequency of Performance*

Task	0 times	1-2 times	3-12 times	13-50 times	51-100 times	100 or more times	No answer
1. Planned and developed individualized instructional programs for other hospital units	46	28	20	5	–	–	1
2. Assisted others in planning and developing individualized instructional programs	25	32	35	7	1	–	–
3. Planned and developed group instructional programs for other hospital units	29	27	32	9	1	1	1
4. Assisted others in planning and developing group instructional programs	15	28	42	13	2	–	–
5. Planned or developed instructional materials for other hospital units	31	24	35	7	1	–	2
6. Assisted others in developing instructional materials	13	28	41	14	2	1	1
7. Evaluated education and training machinery and equipment and recommended purchase	8	25	52	12	2	1	–
8. Evaluated education and training materials and recommended purchase	7	17	47	24	3	2	–
9. Made available a variety of education and training resources for the use of others in the hospital	4	10	35	30	11	9	1

Frequency (N=587)

(continued on next page)

TABLE 7. *(continued)*

	Frequency (N=587)						
Task	0 times	1-2 times	3-12 times	13-50 times	51-100 times	100 or more times	No answer
10. Recommended training and education to resolve specific performance problems in the hospital	6	20	57	14	2	1	—
11. Counseled hospital employees regarding education and training related to their career goals or work problems	8	11	37	31	8	5	—

TABLE 8. *Percent of Educators Who Taught Courses One or More Times Per Year, by Rank Order of Subject Area Taught*

Rank Order	Subject Area	Percent Who Taught (N = 561)*
1.0	Nursing	59
2.0	Management and supervisory development	51
3.0	Other areas	23
4.5	Orientation	17
4.5	Fire, safety, disaster	17
6.0	Education	13
7.5	Patient education	10
7.5	Labor relations	10
9.5	Finance	6
9.5	Death and dying	6

*Twenty-six, or 4 percent, of the 587 respondents indicated that they had not taught during the past year.

Evaluation

Educators were active in evaluating educational materials and programs, as Table 9 indicates. Talking informally with department heads and administration to determine the effectiveness of education and training was the most frequently reported task in this category, with 96 percent of the respondents participating. Forty-six percent of the respondents performed the task from 3 to 12 times during the past year, and 29 percent, from 13 to 50 times.

Advancing the Cause of Education

The frequency with which the respondents performed three tasks related to advancing the cause of education is shown in Table 10. One-half of the respondents informed institutional management and administration of new developments in education and training from 3 to 12 times during the past year; 40 percent gave talks or speeches to various groups regarding hospital education and training with the same frequency. Thirty-nine percent prepared and distributed promotional materials to the hospital staff from 13 to 50 times during the past year.

Managing Facilities

Table 11 indicates that the majority of the respondents spent some time managing educational facilities, although no clear frequency pattern emerged for any of the four tasks in this category.

Establishing and Maintaining Relations with Other Organizations

It is common practice for educators in health care institutions to establish and to maintain relations with other organizations such as governmental agencies and educational institutions, and the respondents participating in this survey were no exception. Table 12 shows that the majority performed each of the first three tasks in this category between 1 and 12 times during the past year.

Personal Professional Development

The educators' interest in their personal professional development is reflected in Table 13. All respondents spent some time reading books, magazines, journals, and catalogs for background information; 58 percent performed this task 51 or more times during the past year. One-half of the respondents attended meetings of professional associations, such as ASHET, the American Society for Training and Development (ASTD), or the American Nurses' Association (ANA), between 3 and 12 times; 62 percent attended educational activities outside the hospital for their personal professional development between 13 and 50 times.

TABLE 9. *Percent of Educators Who Performed Educational Evaluation Tasks, by Frequency of Performance*

Task	Frequency (N=587)						
	0 times	1-2 times	3-12 times	13-50 times	51-100 times	100 or more times	No answer
1. Developed criteria against which training and education materials and/or programs can be evaluated	20	32	36	9	–	1	2
2. Assisted others in developing criteria against which training and education materials or programs can be evaluated	29	32	31	6	1	–	1
3. Designed evaluation instruments and/or activities for training and education materials or programs	18	33	39	7	1	1	1
4. Assisted others in designing evaluation instruments or activities for training and education materials or programs	27	35	31	6	–	–	1
5. Talked informally with department heads and administration to determine the effectiveness of education and training	4	16	46	29	3	2	–

TABLE 10. *Percent of Educators Who Performed Tasks to Advance the Cause of Education, by Frequency of Performance*

Task	Frequency (N=587)						
	0 times	1-2 times	3-12 times	13-50 times	51-100 times	100 or more times	No answer
1. Prepared and distributed notices, bulletins, newsletters, or other promotional materials to hospital staff	7	5	19	39	17	13	–
2. Gave talks or speeches to various groups regarding hospital education and training	18	28	40	10	3	1	–
3. Informed management and administration of new developments in education and training	9	20	50	17	3	1	–

TABLE 11. *Percent of Educators Who Performed Tasks Regarding Educational Facilities Management, by Frequency of Performance*

Task	Frequency (N=587)						
	0 times	1-2 times	3-12 times	13-50 times	51-100 times	100 or more times	No answer
1. Requested alterations of the physical plant for the education and training unit	23	44	29	4	–	–	–
2. Planned the arrangement or rearrangement of education and training department space, furniture, and equipment to meet changing work requirements	18	40	33	6	1	2	–
3. Requisitioned special equipment and furnishings for education and training unit	14	34	42	8	1	1	–
4. Scheduled use of education and training facilities and equipment	11	8	17	30	16	17	1

TABLE 12. *Percent of Educators Who Performed Tasks to Establish and Maintain Relations with Other Organizations, by Frequency of Performance*

Task	Frequency (N=587)						
	0 times	1-2 times	3-12 times	13-50 times	51-100 times	100 or more times	No answer
1. Coordinated training and education unit work with other agencies (i.e., educational institutions, government agencies)	14	18	42	19	5	2	–
2. Developed proposals for federal or foundation projects	26	16	35	18	4	1	–
3. Represented hospital at meetings with other agencies or organizations	14	18	42	19	5	2	–
4. Arranged for hospital employees to attend education and training activities outside of the hospital	13	10	35	29	8	5	–

TABLE 13. *Percent of Educators Who Performed Tasks Regarding Personal Professional Development, by Frequency of Performance*

Task	Frequency (N=587)						
	0 times	1-2 times	3-12 times	13-50 times	51-100 times	100 or more times	No answer
1. Read books, magazines, journals, and catalogs for background information on education and training	–	–	6	35	25	33	–
2. Attended meetings of professional organizations (e.g., ASHET, ASTD, ANA)	7	13	50	27	2	1	–
3. Attended education and training activities outside the hospital for my personal development	–	2	14	62	18	2	2

A Variety of Tasks

The frequency with which the educators performed a variety of tasks did not form a pattern. A majority of the respondents performed 72 of the 74 tasks at least once during the past year. Sixty-six percent did not mediate disagreements among managers of other organizational units, and 62 percent did not type correspondence.

Although it is possible that the frequency intervals used in this survey were too broad or too narrow, there is a more likely explanation of the lack of pattern. First, educators in health care institutions have a wide variety of academic backgrounds. For example, the level of academic achievement ranges from a high school diploma (29 percent) to a doctorate (3 percent). The range of formal studies includes nursing (36 percent), nursing education (11 percent), education (10 percent), liberal arts (8 percent), psychology (5 percent), business administration (4 percent), public health (2 percent), and personnel (1 percent). This diversity suggests that there is a variety of selection-in processes* for the occupation, which probably results in a profession characterized by heterogeneous personality types, intellectual skills, and methods of performing.

Second, the respondents work in institutions that are faced with a variety of environmental constraints and contingencies. For example, inner-city hospitals have manpower problems that are different from those of rural or suburban hospitals. Some health care institutions are unionized, some are not.

Third, because the variety of institutional environments gives rise to differences in the education function within institutions, it is likely that respondents work with mandates that not only are heterogeneous but that also vary considerably in precision and clarity.

Importance of Tasks

The job analysis survey also investigated the respondents' perceptions of the importance of the tasks that they performed. The final question on the survey asked each respondent to list by number the five or fewer tasks that he considered most important to success on the job. The 11

---

*The selection-in process is the series of interactions between personal traits and social phenomena that result in the entrance of some persons into one occupation, to the exclusion of other persons.

tasks most frequently listed are ranked in order in Table 14. Although none of the 74 tasks in the survey received a simple majority, this lack of agreement may be a result of the respondents' being required to select only 5 of 74.

The 11 tasks considered most important fall into three categories: managing the education unit (ranked 1, 6, 7.5[a], and 10.5[a]), providing educational services (ranked 2, 3, 4, 5, and 7.5[b]), and engaging in personal professional development (ranked 9 and 10.5[b]).

It is interesting that 49 percent ranked "preparing a written plan of objectives" as important to success on the job but that only 22 percent believed that examining the work of the unit against this plan was important. Perhaps this indicates that written statements of objectives are perfunctory for education units or that changes in the institutional demands on the units occurred so rapidly that the written plans were outdated before they had been implemented (see task ranked 2). The objectives may have been written in such a manner that they did not aid in implementation. Perhaps achieving the written objectives was not as important as the method by which those objectives were achieved (see tasks ranked 2, 3, 4, and 5).

The tasks ranked 2 through 5 suggest the respondents' attempts to secure agreement with and commitment to the services that they provided. This interpretation is supported by the fact that "talking informally with department heads and administrators to determine the effectiveness of education and training" (ranked 19.5 among tasks selected as important to job success) was the most frequently performed task in the educational evaluation grouping (see Table 9). The importance of securing agreement and commitment should not be surprising, because the answers to such questions as "What should be taught?" "To whom?" and "How?" are necessarily value judgments. Success in providing educational services to employees of health care institutions depends on being responsive to the variety of values held by various persons and groups within the institution.

TABLE 14. *Rank Order of First 11 Tasks Selected as Important to Job Success, by Percent of Respondents Selecting and Percent of Respondents Performing Each Task*

Rank Order	Task Statement	Percent Selecting	Percent Performing
1.0	Prepared a written plan of objectives and priorities for education and training unit	49	95
2.0	Developed training and education activities and/or services in response to requests from department heads or administrative staff	33	95
3.0	Analyzed current hospital problems or interests to determine the need for new training and education programs or changes in existing programs	30	95
4.0	Talked informally with department heads and administrative staff to determine possible education and training activities	25	98
5.0	Conducted carefully planned interviews with department heads, administrative staff, and other personnel to determine possible education and training activities	24	82
6.0	Examined the work of training and education unit in light of established objectives and priorities	22	95
7.5[a]	Prepared suggested budgets covering education and training operations for submission to administration	17	79
7.5[b]	Taught courses	17	94

(continued on next page)

TABLE 14. *(continued)*

Rank Order	Task Statement	Percent Selecting	Percent Performing
9.0	Read books, magazines, journals, and catalogs for background information on education and training	14	99
10.5[a]	Set performance standards for education and training personnel based on organizational priorities	13	67
10.5[b]	Attended education and training activities outside the hospital for my personal development	13	98

Implications for Curriculum

To develop and to maintain integration with a highly differentiated system such as a health care institution, an educator not only must apply knowledge about education and the management of an organization but also must understand and be sensitive to the variety of values held by members of the organization and to the consequent differences in the goals of other units as well as the various means of achieving these goals.

Four terms that are fundamental to this discussion are defined as follows:

- *Understanding* is the ability to comprehend a written, oral, or symbolic communication. Understanding usually involves changing the communication to a meaningful form in one's mind and making simple extensions from it.
- *Analyzing* is breaking down material into its constituent parts and determining the relationship of the parts and the way in which they are organized.
- *Synthesizing* is the process of working with parts of a communication and combining them to create a new pattern or structure.
- *Evaluating* is the ability to use criteria, either given or developed, in order to make judgments.

Based on the findings of the functional job analysis, the following skills appear to be required of educators in health care institutions:

Entry skills
1. Verbal fluency
2. Sensitivity to others
3. Flexibility in adapting to new situations and new persons

Cognitive skills
1. An understanding of the hospital as a social system
   a. Constraints and contingencies presented by community groups and by various governmental agencies
   b. The role of governing boards, medical staff, administration, nursing staff, and so forth
   c. The role of the education unit
      • Clarity of mandate
      • Congruity of goals of education unit with the goals of the hospital
      • Establishing relations with representatives of hospital administration and management
   d. The decision-making process, including the influence structure
   e. Problems of integration and differentiation
   f. Language specific to the hospital

2. An understanding of the relationship between individual behavior and situational variables in an organization
   a. The role of cultural values
   b. Personality and role behavior

3. An understanding of the factors important to the effective utilization of groups as problem-solving and decision-making entities
   a. Group norms
   b. Member functioning
   c. Leadership orientation
   d. Inhibiting and facilitating factors

4. An understanding of the principles and generalizations of behavioral science as they apply to the learning characteristics of students, to instructional procedures, and to teaching

5. An ability to synthesize a plan to generate from a variety of sources appropriate information for educational decision making
   a. Interviewing techniques
   b. Questionnaire development
   c. Test development
   d. Worker observation
   e. Analysis of records and reports

6. An ability to synthesize a plan for educational programs that are acceptable to a variety of clients
   a. Individualized instruction
   b. Group instruction
   c. Mass instruction

7. An ability to analyze and evaluate new contributions to the literature of education and of organizations

The findings of the functional job analysis presented in this report will be used along with other data in the next phase of the Hospitalwide Education and Training Project to develop recommendations for curriculums for educators in health care institutions.

References

1. Schechter, D. S. *Agenda for Continuing Education: A Challenge to Health Care Institutions,* p. 1. Chicago: Hospital Research and Educational Trust, 1974.

2. Tyler, R. W. *Basic Principles of Curriculum and Instruction,* pp. 3-4. Chicago: University of Chicago Press, 1971.

3. Ibid., p. 5.

4. Ibid., pp. 6-33.

5. Flanagan, J. C. The critical incident technique. *Psychol Bull* 51:327, July 1954.

6. Fine, S. A. *The Nature of Jobs and Their Education and Training Requirements,* p. 7. McLean, VA: U.S. Department of Labor, 1964.

7. American Association of School Librarians. *School Library Project.* Chicago: American Library Association, 1971.

8. Technomics, Inc. *Job Analysis Techniques for Restructuring Health Manpower Education and Training.* Springfield, VA: National Technical Information Service, 1972.

9. Center for Occupational and Professional Assessment. *Job Analysis for Selection, Training and Testing of Police Personnel.* Princeton, NJ: Educational Testing Service, 1974.

10. Schechter, *Agenda for Continuing Education,* pp. 12-13.

11. Bloom, B. S. et al. *Taxonomy of Educational Objectives, Handbook I: Cognitive Domain,* pp. 89-176. New York: David McKay Company, Inc., 1956.

Appendix C

Questionnaire
for Health Manpower Educators and Trainers

```
Please return by March 20, 1976
HOSPITAL RESEARCH AND EDUCATIONAL TRUST
840 North Lake Shore Drive
Chicago, Illinois  60611




                              Task Analysis Survey
                    HEALTH MANPOWER EDUCATORS AND TRAINERS
```

```
Please refer to the mailing label above, answer the question below, and
note any additions or corrections.
```

```
Is the information on the
above label correct?
                            Correction(s)

[ ]  Yes        _____

[ ]  No         _____

                _____
```

TASK ANALYSIS SURVEY
HEALTH MANPOWER EDUCATORS AND TRAINERS

SECTION A

1. Please indicate which category best describes your organization.

    ____Health care delivery institution (<u>Please skip to Section B</u>)

    ____Consortium of health care institutions (<u>Please skip to Section C</u>)

    ____Other (Specify)_____

> If you are not employed by a health care delivery
> institution or a consortium of health care institu-
> tions, <u>PLEASE STOP HERE</u> and return this questionnaire.
> The remaining questions are directed only to educators/
> trainers in health care delivery institutions or in
> consortia.

SECTION B

1. What is the size of your health care delivery institution?

    ____Less than 100 beds   ____300 to 399 beds

    ____100 to 199 beds   ____400 to 499 beds

    ____200 to 299 beds   ____500 beds or more

2. Is your institution a member of a consortium for education and training
    activities?

        ____Yes   ____No

3. Is your institution involved in conducting degree or certificate programs in cooperation with <u>educational</u> institutions?

_____Yes   _____No

If "yes", please check the kind(s) of institutions with which you are cooperating.

_____University   _____Vocational-technical School

_____Four-year College   _____High School

_____Two-year College   _____Other (Specify)_____

4. Does your institution have a separate administrative unit with responsibility for education and training activities?

_____Yes   _____No

5. Which of the following best describes the administrative unit in which you work?

_____Education and Training

___Nursing

___Personnel

___Other (Specify)_____

SECTION C

1. How many other health care institutions are members of your consortium?

_____3 or less

_____4 or 5

_____Between 6 and 9

_____10 or more

2. Is an institution(s) of higher education a member of your consortium?

    ____Yes   ____No

If "yes", please specify the type(s) of institutions that hold membership.

    ____University   ____Vocational-technical School

    ____Four-year College   ____High School

    ____Two-year College   ____Other (Specify)_____

PLEASE PROCEED TO SECTION D

SECTION D

1. If you possess one or more college degrees, please specify the two highest degrees and the fields in which they were earned.

             Degree   Field

    _____   _____

    _____   _____

2. What do you consider your major professional field at this time?

    ____Nursing   ____Personnel

    ____Education and Training   ____Other (Specify)_____

3. How long have you held your current position with your present employer?

 ____Less than 1 year

 ____1 year but less than 2 years

 ____2 years but less than 3 years

 ____3 years but less than 5 years

 ____5 years or more

4. How long has this position existed in your institution or consortium?

 ____Less than 1 year

 ____1 year but less than 2 years

 ____2 years but less than 3 years

 ____3 years but less than 5 years

 ____5 years or more

5. What percentage of your time do you spend in the duties of this position?

 ____Less than 25%

 ____25% to 49%

 ____50% to 74%

 ____75% to 100%

6. Would you describe your current position as:

 ____Manager/Director of Education and Training, Health Care Institution

 ____Manager/Director of Consortium

 ____Staff of Education and Training Unit, Health Care Institution

 ____Staff of Education and Training, Consortium

PLEASE PROCEED TO SECTION E

SECTION E The responsibilities of hospital education and training staff vary in different settings. We would like to determine the job content in your institution based on your experience. After reading through the entire list of tasks below, please circle one letter on each line as an estimate of the frequency with which you personally performed the activity during the last year. If you have not performed a specific task, circle the 0 in the first column. Please respond to each statement. Remember that some of the tasks may not be appropriate to your situation.

During the last year I have performed this task approximately:

TASKS	0 times	1 or 2 times	3 to 12 times	13 to 50 times	51 to 100 times	100 or more times
1. Prepared a written plan of objectives and priorities for education and training unit.	a	b	c	d	e	f
2. Examined the work of training and education unit in the light of established objectives and priorities.	a	b	c	d	e	f
3. Reviewed changes in hospital policies and procedures to determine the effect on education and training unit.	a	b	c	d	e	f
4. Adjusted the assignments of training and education personnel to meet work demands.	a	b	c	d	e	f
5. Informed training and education staff of policy or procedural changes which affect their work.	a	b	c	d	e	f

	0 times	1 or 2 times	3 to 12 times	13 to 50 times	51 to 100 times	100 or more times
6. Developed job descriptions for education and training personnel.	a	b	c	d	e	f
7. Set performance standards for training and education personnel based on organizational priorities.	a	b	c	d	e	f
8. Conducted performance appraisals of training and education personnel based on personal knowledge and data relevant to job performance.	a	b	c	d	e	f
9. Made recommendations for promotions, transfers, and salary increases for training and education personnel.	a	b	c	d	e	f
10. Resolved differences among training and education employees.	a	b	c	d	e	f
11. Reviewed program designs and reports prepared by training and education personnel.	a	b	c	d	e	f
12. Conducted education and training unit staff meetings to coordinate activities.	a	b	c	d	e	f
13. Conducted in-service training for training and education personnel.	a	b	c	d	e	f

	0 times	1 or 2 times	3 to 12 times	13 to 50 times	51 to 100 times	100 or more times
14. Interviewed prospective education and training personnel.	a	b	c	d	e	f
15. Selected prospective education and training personnel.	a	b	c	d	e	f
16. Prepared suggested budgets covering education and training operations for submission to administration.	a	b	c	d	e	f
17. Allocated the budget assigned to education and training.	a	b	c	d	e	f
18. Reported to administration expenditures to date.	a	b	c	d	e	f
19. Talked informally with department heads and administrative staff to determine possible education and training activities.	a	b	c	d	e	f
20. Conducted carefully planned interviews with department heads, administrative staff and other personnel to determine possible education and training activities.	a	b	c	d	e	f

	0 times	1 or 2 times	3 to 12 times	13 to 50 times	51 to 100 times	100 or more times
21. Prepared and distributed questionnaires to learn about possible education and training activities.	a	b	c	d	e	f
22. Analyzed the job descriptions of various hospital staff to ascertain possible training and education activities.	a	b	c	d	e	f
23. Analyzed existing organizational policies to determine possible education and training activities.	a	b	c	d	e	f
24. Analyzed hospital or departmental procedure manuals to determine possible education and training activities.	a	b	c	d	e	f
25. Analyzed current hospital problems or interests to determine the need for new training and education programs or changes in existing programs.	a	b	c	d	e	f
26. Analyzed patients' records in the light of staff capabilities to determine education and training activities.	a	b	c	d	e	f

	0 times	1 or 2 times	3 to 12 times	13 to 50 times	51 to 100 times	100 or more times
27. Planned or assisted others in planning task analysis studies to specify skills and knowledge required for various positions.	a	b	c	d	e	f
28. Observed the work of personnel in other organizational units to help determine problems amenable to training.	a	b	c	d	e	f
29. Assisted in the specification of competencies or criteria for various jobs in the hospital.	a	b	c	d	e	f
30. Developed training and education activities and/or services in response to requests from department heads or administrative staff.	a	b	c	d	e	f
31. Recommended training and education to resolve specific performance problems in the hospital.	a	b	c	d	e	f
32. Suggested ways, other than education and training, for dealing with organizational problems.	a	b	c	d	e	f

	0 times	1 or 2 times	3 to 12 times	13 to 50 times	51 to 100 times	100 or more times
33. Assisted others in setting up new systems, writing procedure manuals and the like.	a	b	c	d	e	f
34. Served as a member of hospital committees						
a. To review various hospital policies.	a	b	c	d	e	f
b. To establish hospital budget priorities.	a	b	c	d	e	f
c. To resolve specific hospital problems.	a	b	c	d	e	f
35. Assisted the administrative staff in planning decision-making meetings.	a	b	c	d	e	f
36. Conducted or served as mediator in decision-making meetings.	a	b	c	d	e	f
37. Mediated differences among managers of other organizational units.	a	b	c	d	e	f
38. Planned and developed individualized instructional programs for other hospital units.	a	b	c	d	e	f
39. Planned and developed group instructional programs for other hospital units.	a	b	c	d	e	f

	0 times	1 or 2 times	3 to 12 times	13 to 50 times	51 to 100 times	100 or more times
40. Assisted others in planning and developing individualized instructional programs.	a	b	c	d	e	f
41. Assisted others in planning and developing group instructional programs.	a	b	c	d	e	f
42. Planned or develop instructional material for other hospital units.	a	b	c	d	e	f
43. Assisted others in developing instructional material.	a	b	c	d	e	f
44. Taught courses in: (Please list)	a	b	c	d	e	f
_____	a	b	c	d	e	f
_____	a	b	c	d	e	f
_____	a	b	c	d	e	f
_____	a	b	c	d	e	f
45. Developed criteria against which training and education materials and/or programs can be evaluated.	a	b	c	d	e	f

	0 times	1 or 2 times	3 to 12 times	13 to 50 times	51 to 100 times	100 or more times
46. Assisted others in developing criteria against which training and education materials or programs can be evaluated.	a	b	c	d	e	f
47. Designed evaluation instruments and/or activities for training and education materials or programs.	a	b	c	d	e	f
48. Assisted others in designing evaluation instruments or activities for training and education materials or programs.	a	b	c	d	e	f
49. Talked informally with department heads and administration to determine the effectiveness of education and training.	a	b	c	d	e	f
50. Developed a system for recording data about the education and training of employees of the organization.	a	b	c	d	e	f
51. Maintained such a system.	a	b	c	d	e	f
52. Prepared written reports for administration and/or other managers about the education and training of employees.	a	b	c	d	e	f

	0 times	1 or 2 times	3 to 12 times	13 to 50 times	51 to 100 times	100 or more times
53. Prepared and distributed notices, bulletins, newsletters or other promotional materials to hospital staff.	a	b	c	d	e	f
54. Gave talks or speeches to various groups regarding hospital education and training.	a	b	c	d	e	f
55. Informed management and administration of new developments in education and training.	a	b	c	d	e	f
56. Evaluated education and training machinery and equipment and recommended purchase.	a	b	c	d	e	f
57. Evaluated education and training materials and recommended purchase.	a	b	c	d	e	f
58. Made available a variety of education and training resources for the use of others in the hospital.	a	b	c	d	e	f
59. Counseled hospital employees regarding education and training related to their career goals or work related problems.	a	b	c	d	e	f

	0 times	1 or 2 times	3 to 12 times	13 to 50 times	51 to 100 times	100 or more times
60. Arranged for hospital employees to attend education and training activities outside of the hospital.	a	b	c	d	e	f
61. Requested alterations of the physical plant for the education and training unit.	a	b	c	d	e	f
62. Planned the arrangement or rearrangement of education and training department space, furniture, and equipment to meet changing work requirements.	a	b	c	d	e	f
63. Requisitioned special equipment and furnishings for education and training unit.	a	b	c	d	e	f
64. Scheduled use of education and training facilities and equipment.	a	b	c	d	e	f
65. Coordinated training and education unit work with other agencies (i.e. educational institutions, government agencies).	a	b	c	d	e	f
66. Developed proposals for federal or foundation projects.	a	b	c	d	e	f

	0 times	1 or 2 times	3 to 12 times	13 to 50 times	51 to 100 times	100 or more times
67. Represented hospital at meetings with other agencies or organizations.	a	b	c	d	e	f
68. Read books, magazines, journals, catalogs for background information on education and training.	a	b	c	d	e	f
69. Attended meetings of professional organizations (e.g. ASHET, ASTD, ANA).	a	b	c	d	e	f
70. Attended education and training activities outside the hospital for my personal development.	a	b	c	d	e	f
71. Initiated or responded to correspondence regarding training and education department procedures, activities and services.	a	b	c	d	e	f
72. Typed correspondence.	a	b	c	d	e	f

SECTION F

1. From the 72 tasks listed in Section **E**, please list by number the five
   (or fewer) that you consider <u>most</u> important to success in your job.

        a. _____   c. _____

        b. _____   d. _____

                e. _____